The Original Works of
EUNICE D. INGHAM

Stories the Feet Can Tell Thru Reflexology

Stories the Feet Have Told Thru Reflexology

WITH REVISIONS BY DWIGHT C. BYERS

INGHAM PUBLISHING, INC. • PUBLISHER
Saint Petersburg • Florida U.S.A.

ISBN 0-9611804-3-9
Revised Edition, 1984
Sixth Printing, 1996

Published and Distributed Throughout the World by

INGHAM PUBLISHING, INC. • PUBLISHER
Post Office Box 12642
Saint Petersburg, Florida 33733-2642, U.S.A.

Printed in the United States of America

This publication contains the combined works of Eunice D. Ingham (Stopfel), developer of the science of Reflexology. The original text is reprinted with some clarifying revisions by Dwight C. Byers, nephew of Eunice Ingham. The purpose of this combined version is to provide readers with one easy-to-follow reference to the ORIGINAL INGHAM METHOD™ by making all the information of the two books accessible under one cover.

As a follow-up in your study of the ORIGINAL INGHAM METHOD™, read "Better Health With Foot Reflexology" (including Hand Reflexology) by Dwight C. Byers, President of the International Institute of Reflexology. This book is the most concise, up-to-date guide to Reflexology available today. To obtain this book, seminar information, charts or any of our other materials, write to:

Ingham Publishing, Inc.
International Institute of Reflexology
P.O. Box 12642
St. Petersburg, Florida 33733-2642 U.S.A.

Stories The Feet Can Tell

CONTENTS

Stories The Feet Have Told

CONTENTS

STORIES

THE FEET

CAN TELL

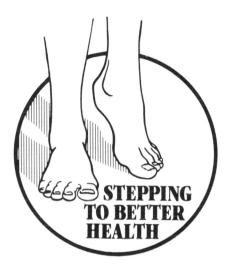

STEPPING
TO BETTER
HEALTH

REFLEXOLOGY

By
EUNICE D. INGHAM

How beautiful upon the mountains are the feet of him that bringeth good tidings.

ISAIAH 52:7

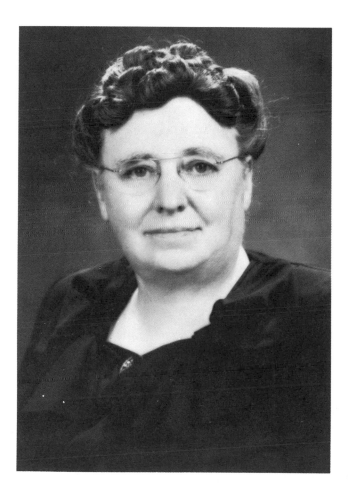

Author and Lecturer
EUNICE D. INGHAM STOPFEL
Feb. 24, 1889 — Dec. 10, 1974

Preface

As author of this little book, I will endeavor to bring to light and explain the actual location of the various reflexes in the feet, as discovered by a careful study in my practice as a physiotherapist, with hundreds of patients, with whom I have had astonishing results.

Founder of Zone Therapy

Dr. Wm. H. Fitzgerald, founder of ZONE THERAPY, held a position that commands respect. He was a graduate of the University of Vermont, and spent two and one-half years in the Boston City Hospital. He was a member of the staff in the Central London Nose and Throat Hospital, and for two years he was in Vienna, where he was assistant to Professor Politzer and Professor Otto Chiari, who are known wherever medical textbooks are read.

While head of the Nose and Throat Department of St. Francis Hospital, Hartford, Conn., his discovery of the Chinese method of ZONE THERAPY was brought to the attention of the medical world, pointing out the fact that pressure, and the massaging of certain zones, has a definite effect in bringing about normal physiological functioning in all parts of the zone treated, no matter how remote this area may be from the part upon which the treatment is exerted.

Dr. Fitzgerald, in his work entitled ZONE THERAPY, blazes the path for these further developments as he brings to light for our consideration his discovery of the ten various zones of the body and location of each organ in the body in one or more of these zones.

I want to mention here that I owe a debt of gratitude for my success in this field, to my great teacher, Joe S. Riley, M.D., and his wife, whose names are familiar to many of you as pioneers in the field of ZONE THERAPY.

It was my privilege to be associated with them for several years in their general practice, during which time the methods which will be described in this book, were successfully practiced on hundreds of patients who visited his office.

Each reflex and point of contact has been carefully and thoughtfully checked and rechecked, until with all confidence we call your attention to these findings, sincerely trusting they will prove helpful and beneficial to others.

I hope that these following pages may prove to be another stepping stone to greater heights along this new but effective way of helping those who seek for better health and efficiency.

EUNICE D. INGHAM

Introduction

The foundation theory of this work as set forth in the following pages has been built up entirely on the opinions of practicing physicians who have had the opportunity of observing the remarkable results obtained from this particular form of reflex therapy.

So let me say should anyone, physician or layman, after a careful study and application of this method, have any valuable suggestions in the form of an explanation to offer, I will be glad to hear from them. Like every new development, it must prove its efficiency to many a doubting skeptic, before being accepted as an established fact.

Many of you will remember, not so long ago, the attitude manifested when the X-ray was first brought to the attention of the world. Yet today it is acknowledged by all as a most valuable asset to the success of the medical profession. We learn from the work of Dr. John C. Hemmeter entitled "Master Minds in Medicine" that it was not until toward the end of the sixteenth century that intellectual Europe was ripe for the acceptance of the discovery of the circulation of the blood. Dr. Michael Servetus planted the seed—Dr. Columbo watered it and to Dr. William Harvey remained the troublesome work of the harvest. And what we possess today in knowledge of the circulation of the blood, we possess through him who, armed only with a magnifying glass, accomplished such great things in spite of bitter criticism.

Stories the Feet
Can Tell

I have chosen the unique title, "Stories the Feet Can Tell," for my work because I believe it is possible to learn many a valuable story from the use of Foot Reflexology. A careful study and application of the methods as described and set forth in the following pages and illustrations, may reveal many a hidden secret of some weakness here or there that may not be manifesting itself yet in any serious degree.

Perhaps a sluggish liver is responsible for the trouble in the intestinal tract that results in constipation. Can the feet be made to tell the story so that the cause of that constipation may be found? Let us see if we find the nerve endings in the right foot reflexing to the liver very tender. If so we know there is a crystal-like formation there interfering with the circulation of the blood to the liver, preventing it from functioning normally. As we work this out we are giving nature a chance to carry away the waste matter and restore the normal circulation to the affected part or parts.

1

You can readily see how necessary it is that we keep the chemical balance of our blood stream normal and free from crystalline deposits so the feet will have no serious stories to tell. We are all familiar with what the effect of sand or gravel would be in a garden hose, yet we expect our body to function properly regardless of obstructions in the delicate nerve endings.

We forget that our body is supposed to contain about 22 X miles of tubing. Every inch of this tubing is kept in activity by contraction and relaxation, dependent entirely upon the muscular activity of the individual. Thus we can see the benefit of any form of therapy or exercise that might increase the circulation and strengthen the action of our muscles.

No matter what line of healing you may follow at the present time keep this book at hand, and where others fail to bring about the desired results, try this simple method of producing a reflex action (by manipulation) through the nerve endings on the soles of the feet.

A few case records are given in this book to emphasize the results that have been obtained, which are in no way overdrawn or overestimated. I am enthusiastic only to the extent of the success I have already obtained in my own experience as a physiotherapist.

And now with the very best wishes for the success of every one who is willing to try it out, I will pass on and explain to the best of my ability, the exact reflex method to be used in the treatment of various ailments.

Don't let the common mistake of its simplicity rob it of any importance. The why and wherefore I am not prepared to explain, I only ask that you try it out. My sincere wish is that every one will become proficient and successful in this great work.

Perfect Health Spells
Perfect Feet

As soon as we allow the muscles of our body to weaken, the muscle tissue in our feet gives way. The body structure goes down and one or more of the twenty-six bones in each foot may become misplaced causing undue pressure on some nerve ending. This shuts off a certain portion of the normal nerve and blood supply in the bottom of the feet, and as any part of the blood stream becomes choked, it slows down the circulation. As the result of this slowing down of the circulation we have a formation of chemical deposits or waste matter forming in and around the misplaced joints.

While this condition remains in the feet it is diagnosed as broken arches. Let it exist long enough and finally we discover trouble in another part of the body. If this obstruction happens to be in the nerve endings or reflex leading to the kidneys, we find the kidneys are being robbed of a part of their blood supply. This in turn interferes with the proper contraction and relaxation that is necessary in order that the kidneys may carry on their part of eliminating the uric acid from the system. The more of these deposits that have formed, the longer we will have to work these reflexes to dissolve them so that nature can carry away and dispose of this waste matter. This restores the normal circulation to the one or more organs involved.

Again we find another cause for a formation of waste matter or crystal-like formation in the nerve endings where the construction of every bone and muscle of the foot is apparently normal. Perhaps we have inherited or otherwise acquired a certain weakness of some part or organ of the body. The normal muscular activity of that organ is lessened and its function of contraction and relaxing is interfered with. So there has not been sufficient force of circulation to keep that nerve ending free and clear.

3

A misplaced vertebra, in any part of the spine, will be sure to cut off the normal circulation and interfere with the contracting and relaxing of the part which is depending upon this particular nerve for its blood supply.

Where this may be the cause, we find the corresponding location in the spinal reflexes, as shown in Fig. 5, very tender, but by applying plenty of this Reflexology method to the reflex leading to this vertebra, we will be sure to help nature repair whatever may have gone haywire. In studying a chart of the nervous system we can see how utterly dependent it is upon the spine for its blood supply; even the slightest undue pressure in any part of the spine cannot help but interfere with the contracting and relaxing process necessary to keep the nerve endings of the feet to that part involved free from any crystalline deposits.

Our body is said to be sixty percent fluid. How necessary it is to have this flowing through the tissue in a healthy condition and not overburdened with poisonous acid.

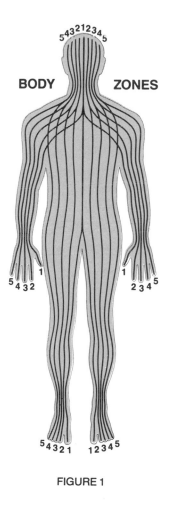

BODY   ZONES

FIGURE 1

A study of this diagram will graphically place in the mind the zones of the body.

As there are ten fingers and toes, we may conceive ten zones of the limbs and all parts of the body.

Zone Therapy

Now when you proceed with this Chinese method of ZONE THERAPY and begin with the firm pressure of your thumb to examine the reflexes of the feet, you will soon determine the location of the trouble that is sending out the danger signal. Your patients will be amazed that you find such sore places which they had no idea could possibly be found on their feet, since no trouble in the form of any foot discomfort had ever manifested itself in any way to them.

Then again we hear people say, "Oh, my feet hurt, I am sick all over," yet little attention is given by them to see if these pains or disturbances felt at various times might be a warning of a new weakness here or there, not yet manifested in any other part of the body.

A CORN HERE AND CALLOUS THERE

They try one shoe after another, one hurting here and one hurting there. They visit various Podiatrists who are caring scientifically for many minor foot ills to which mankind is heir. Yet their trouble continues, a corn here, a callous there, to impede the natural source of circulation. Yet little do they realize that this undue pressure on some important nerve ending may result in possible injury to each organ dependent upon this particular source for its nerve energy.

This work being the outcome of my study of ZONE THERAPY, I have been granted permission by Dr. J. S. Riley to use his chart on Zone Markings for the purpose of giving you an idea of the ten zones of our body and how to locate them.

TEN ZONES

As you will see, we have ten fingers and ten toes, our whole organism being divided into ten zones. From a study of the chart, Fig. 1, you can readily see what we mean by the ten zones of our body. Each line is drawn through the center of its respective zone, and the entire zone includes all parts and organs through which the respective zone line passes.

The right and left sides of the body are the same and each zone passes through the body from front to back, or from back to front. This is true of the legs and arms, also the feet and hands.

LOCATING THE ZONES

Take any of the internal organs of the body, and determine what zone lines pass through them according to the chart. Then picture in your mind on what part of the foot this line will be found and this will guide you somewhat in finding the desired reflex. It is neither hard nor difficult and will only require a little study and practice to make you as proficient as any one in determining the location to be manipulated for any ailment. The fact that it all seems so simple will in no way take away or prevent you from obtaining results. Allow me to say, and emphasize it too, your persistent efforts will be rewarded by many a happy surprise by following the technique found in "Stories The Feet Can Tell."

Reactions Manifested

In giving this treatment, you will find that the intensity of the pain will be in direct proportion to the amount and possibly the size of the crystals, and the length of time these crystals have been accumulating. Now as we continue this Reflex therapy directly over the tender place for a period of one to two minutes, we are rubbing or grinding, these small sharp needle-like crystals into the muscle tissue and almost invariably the second and third treatment will be even more painful than the first. At each treatment we are causing an acceleration of the circulation of the blood through the affected parts, thus increasing the vitality and endurance of the patient. The irritation set up by these crystals naturally causes a reaction.

VARIATIONS IN REACTIONS

It will be interesting to note the variation of reactions in different patients. Just as no two persons react the same to any condition or circumstance in life, just so will each one have a different reaction although seemingly suffering from the same ailment. For this reason, you must use your own judgement in the length of time given to each treatment, and just how frequently the treatments are to be given. Keep in mind first and uppermost what you are doing. You are stimulating the circulation, and as you stimulate the circulation you raise the body vitality, and as the vitality increases, nature has the strength to overcome and throw off the poisons in the system.

The more of this toxic material the blood contains, the more severe will be the reaction. Many times it manifests itself in the form of a severe cold. This is nature's way of cleaning house and eliminating the poisons from the system. Sometimes this happens after the first treatment, but usually it is the second or third treatment that produces this desired effect. If one has a tendency to respond quickly to any form of treatment, the sooner the reaction takes place, just that much sooner will an improvement in the condition be realized from these treatments. I consider it impossible to fully realize, or to in any way estimate, the amount of good that may be accomplished in various cases by work of this kind.

It is here you must remember the possibility of being too severe. If the patient is nervous and high strung, with extremely sensitive reflexes, you must use only a slight pressure at first. Do not give the treatment too often; never more than twice a week in a case of this type.

Reflexes Present in the Hands and Feet

These same reflexes exist in our hands in the same proportion, location, etc., as in our feet. Only it is more difficult to locate them for they are not so pronounced, and the added amount of exercise we give our hands keeps the tenderness worked out, which would otherwise be found.

Our foot we carefully preserve in a shoe, which prevents a certain amount of the natural motion of the foot that would take place if we were constantly walking barefoot in the primitive way nature intended us to follow.

It is estimated that the average pair of feet lift for their owner a total of at least ten cars of coal in weight daily. We forget all this and then wonder why so many people today complain of foot discomfort.

Nature intended that we should walk, bend, twist our feet, and also run occasionally to keep a fresh supply of blood, with the normal circulation surging through every minute joint and nerve extremity of our feet.

But if we allow an excess acid condition to form in our blood stream, we increase the calcium deposits. Then acid crystals, similar to particles of frost when examined under microscope, form in these nerve endings, thus impeding the normal circulation of the blood to the various parts of the body.

CONSTANT MOTION

Our whole body is constantly in motion; the Lungs, Heart, Liver, Kidneys, Intestines, etc. These, when in a perfectly healthy condition, are constantly, day and night, performing their respective duties.

The natural muscular activity of each organ does its part to see that its whole nerve canal is kept free from any detrimental obstruction. But if any one of these members becomes sluggish, weak or injured in any way, it slows down its normal muscular activity to the extent that the extremities of these nerve endings will become clogged. Although only obstructed to a slight degree, yet it may be sufficient to impede the circulation as it returns to supply that organ again with a fresh supply of blood.

It is by the pressure of the thumb coming in contact with these crystals at the nerve endings that causes the pain felt so keenly at these reflexes during the treatment. As they become dissolved by this process the blood carries them away gradually as it makes its circuit to the feet and back to the heart at the rate of about three times a minute.

Let the reflex work be given with a slow forward creeping motion, not using the flat ball of the thumb as much as the corner toward the end. Let the pressure be firm, but at the same time, gently at first and gradually increased with as much as you see the patient is able to endure. The thumb nails must be filed comparatively low. You will often be called upon to prove that it is not your thumb nail causing this pressure on these nerve endings where there is a formation of crystalline deposits. Remember, it is important to keep your eye on the expression of your patient. This will tell you the instant your thumb comes in contact with the irritated crystal-filled nerve endings.

Location of Reflexes

As you sit facing your patient, who is reclining on a couch or table somewhat higher than the stool or chair you will occupy, place the left foot in your right hand; holding the foot firmly. Then with your left hand between the thumb and first finger, clasp the smallest part of the foot, which will be about midway between the base of the toes and lower part of the heel.

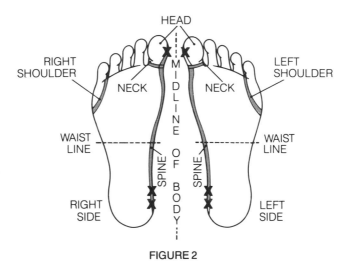

FIGURE 2

This will represent the waist line of the body as shown in Fig. 2. In exact proportion as the organs are located in the body on the left side, above or below this line, the reflex will be found on the sole of the left foot affecting the various parts in the left side of the body. The right foot reflects for the right side in the same proportion. Thus, we find the heart reflected in the left foot, the liver in the right, etc. We have two kidneys, so each foot has a reflex to the kidney on that particular side; the right on the right foot; the left on the left foot.

The ascending colon reflex is on the right foot, as is the right half of the transverse colon, as it traverses the abdomen from right to left just below the liver, stomach and spleen, at about the waist line of the body to the left hypochondriac region on the left side, where it curves downward beneath the lower end of the spleen. Here it is known as the descending colon. This will reflect on the left foot from where it leaves the center of the body.

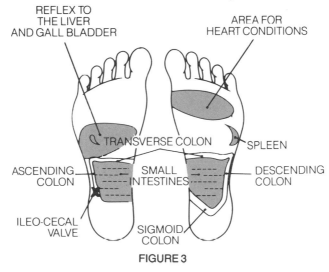

FIGURE 3

For instance, a patient with trouble in the colon, or even a lazy colon, will flinch at the slightest pressure at this point of the waist line of the foot. Now to determine if one part of the colon might be affected more than the other, begin with a firm pressure of the left thumb, just above the heel and on the right foot as shown in Figure 3. Press each portion firmly up the side to the center and across at the waistline of the foot as we have just explained. Then proceed to the other foot and continue the same line of procedure from the inner center line to the side of the left foot and down on the left side following the course of the descending colon in the body.

The point where the greatest amount of tenderness is found will determine the location of the greatest amount of congestion, and where congestion exists disease will result.

THE APPENDIX

You will recall the location of the appendix and how it is situated at the lower border of the ascending colon on the right side. It is a narrow blind-ended worm-like tube from three to six inches long and held in no set position. Since it is in the right side and below the waist line of the body, just so will you find the reflex to this little organ below the waist line of the right foot, toward the edge, just above the round part of the heel, as shown in Fig. 4.

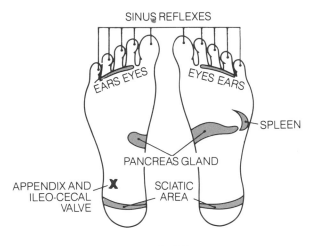

FIGURE 4

If there is any tendency to a congestion of the appendix, it will show up with a tenderness at this point as you apply a firm pressure with your right thumb. But with a few treatments it can usually be worked out.

I have had marvelous results, in a number of cases, where it seemed almost certain that an operation would be necessary for any relief. One particular case I recall where Mr. P. had already been taken from his work to the hospital for the operation. He finally persuaded the physician to allow him to return home and seek relief with this particular form of therapy on the reflex of the foot.

The work was carefully directed under the physician's care. When the tenderness in the reflex on the foot had completely disappeared, the discomfort and pain in the region of the appendix had cleared up and to the present time Mr. P. is working every day and feeling fine. (This does not imply that an acute case would not require the attention of a competent physician.)

ILEO-CECAL VALVE

In almost the same location as the appendix we have what is known as the Ileo-cecal Valve. Fig. 4. This forms the opening from the small intestines into the colon, opening toward the large intestine and guarding against reflex from the large into the small bowel. As to whether the appendix or the Ileo-cecal valve is affected will be hard to determine since the location of both is so nearly alike.

Now if the trouble is in that side, and by working out this tenderness we can cause the symptoms to disappear, you need not worry whether it was the appendix or the little valve that was on a strike at the time it was causing the disturbance. If you get results and bring about relief, you are doing all that is expected of you.

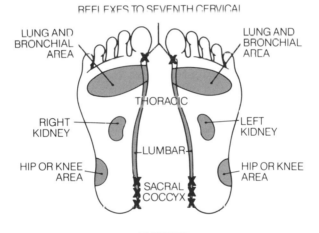

FIGURE 5

When the irritated crystal-filled nerve-endings are stimulated, the corresponding organ which if reflexly connected with this particular sensitive nerve receives an added supply of lifegiving blood. The congested tissue is thus relieved, and the healing process is hastened.

SMALL INTESTINES

For the small intestines, the reflexes are found above the heel line and below the waistline of each foot. Since the small intestines lie in a part of each of the first, second, third, and fourth zones, we must look for them all the way across from the inside almost to the outside of the foot, the right half of the intestines showing on the right foot, and the left half on the left foot. Fig. 3.

STOMACH REFLEXES

The stomach is located just a little above the waist line of the body, almost in the center but a little more to the left side. We find its reflex above the waist line of the foot in the first, second and third zones on the right foot, and the first, second, third and fourth zones of the left foot.

LUNGS AND BRONCHIAL TUBES

The lungs and bronchial tubes being on each side alike will be found in the same location on each foot, a little below the base of the toes. Fig. 5.

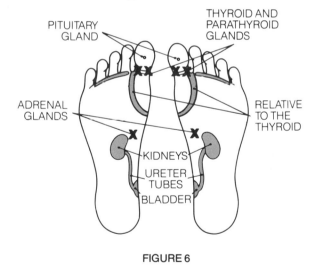

FIGURE 6

PNEUMONIA

Keep this in mind if you are called upon to render relief in case of pneumonia, also the position pictured in Fig. 21. Working the reflexes at this point will relieve a certain amount of tension which is always helpful in pneumonia. In an acute case let no other reflex be worked without the physician's advice.

GALL BLADDER

This being imbedded in the liver, just off center on the right side, you will find its reflex on the right foot deep in, a little under the ball of the foot as shown in Fig. 3.

KIDNEYS

Each kidney will be reflexed in the second and third zone of each foot, at about the waist line of the foot. Fig. 6.

EYES AND EARS

Location and position for reaching the reflex to the eyes and ears given in Fig. 4 and Fig. 7 reaching down from the top onto the foot at the base of the toes.

BLADDER

Location given in Fig. 6 and Fig. 27. Since the bladder is located in the center of the body we will find the reflex in the first zone on the inside of each ankle.

THE SPLEEN

Shape and Location

The Spleen is a soft, brittle, very vascular, oblong, flattened organ embracing the fundus of the stomach, to which it is attached by the gastro-splenic omentum. This completely invests the spleen except at the helium, and where the suspensory ligament is attached.

Its external surface is convex, smooth, and in contact with the under surface on the diaphragm which separates it from the ninth, tenth, and eleventh ribs of the left side. In size and weight it is liable to extreme variations at different periods of life. In the adult it is usually above five inches in length, three or four inches in breadth, and an inch and a half in thickness, and weighs about seven ounces.

SPLEEN AND THE ZONES
Where Located

This description gives you an idea of the zones in which the spleen is located, so you will have no trouble in locating the reflex in the left foot. Remember its location in regard to the waist line of the body and how it will compare to that of your thumb on the nerve reflex to the spleen. See Fig. 4.

I will not say that you can always determine if this tenderness may mean trouble only in the spleen, for we have other important points of contact so close to that of the spleen.

Lying almost in front of the spleen is the splenic flexure, where the transverse colon passes just in front and below the spleen at the left hypochondriac region where it makes its curve downward beneath the lower end of the spleen. Trouble in this particular part of the colon is very often the case.

SPLEEN OR COLON
Which is Wrong?

But if the patient is inclined to be anemic and has already been diagnosed as such by a physician, and you find a tenderness at this point, you can be sure it is the spleen and not the colon that is in need of your attention. It is possible that both conditions might exist, but one thing is certain, you will be able to remedy the trouble, whatever is wrong, by removing those acid crystals from the nerve endings and supplying the parts with the normal circulation.

REPLACING OLD CELLS WITH NEW

Should the trouble be pernicious anemia, it will take longer to obtain results, so do not be too impatient. It takes time to completely replace new cells in any organ of our body.

Therefore, we must wait till nature has exchanged the old for a new model machine before we can look for perfect performance. Do not expect a "model T Ford" compete with a new Cadillac.

ANEMIC CONDITIONS

I cannot recall a single case of simple anemia where this particular point was not extremely tender, for it is the spleen that manufactures the red blood cells. If this spleen fails to do its work through any means of congestion cutting down its blood supply, in turn it will fail to reproduce the substantial red blood cells necessary for our well-being. The spleen is also the burying ground of the old broken down blood cells which by the laws of nature rise again. They are buried and yet they are manufactured there. Nature takes the old and converts them into the new red blood cells.

DIET BENEFICIAL

It is well to remember that a blood building diet is extremely important in overcoming anemic conditions, let this be directed by a competent nutritionist and combined with this special form of Reflexology and your efforts will be rewarded with remarkable results.

19

Eyes

We find a big majority of individuals today whose eyesight is affected in one way or another, perhaps nothing more than astigmatism, a slight flattening of the eyeball, or some condition that could be easily corrected by the wearing of glasses.

SOME CASES INCURABLE

Again we have the poor unfortunate souls who have inherited some form of an infection that can never be wiped out. We do not profess to say that any of these can be benefited by this or any other method, but we do find that some conditions can be greatly improved, even to a form of glaucoma, which is a condition where the eyeballs become very hard. It is produced by the fluids forming in quantities beyond the normal, and thus extending the coats of the eye until excessive strain and hardness are felt, with partial or total blindness.

CASE RECORD
Successful With Glaucoma

One particular case I had of this type was seemingly, to all appearance and according to the doctor's diagnosis, cleared up entirely.

Mr. S., a man about 45 years of age, had become extremely discouraged when informed by several specialists that it would be only a matter of time till his sight would be entirely gone. He was advised not to read or tax his eyes in any way unnecessarily in order to prolong the sight he now had.

By examining his feet I found no tenderness at any point except at the reflex to the eyes, which is found between the second and third toe at the point where they are joined to the foot, and a little below, reaching down, as we might say, from the top of the toes as shown in Fig. 7 and Fig. 4.

We will consider you are working on the left foot, and always have the patient facing you. Now grasp the outside of the foot with your right hand, place your thumb on the sole of the foot, bracing it from the top with your fingers, and with your right thumb reach down from the root of the toes on to the foot in a way to reach the reflex deep down

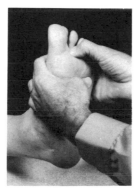

FIGURE 7

**Best Position for Reaching the Reflex
to the Eyes and Ears.**

between and around the base of the second and third toes. It may be necessary to use your finger on the right hand to find the exact location. At least don't give up till you have most thoroughly tried with both hands. It may be necessary for you to reverse the procedure outlined; holding the foot in your right hand and using the thumb and first finger of your left hand to reach these reflexes.

21

This reflex method was carried on persistently, every day, in the case of glaucoma with Mr. S. just mentioned. I was able to see him but once a week, as he lived in a distant city, so I carefully instructed Mrs. S. to follow my direction faithfully by working this reflex every day.

After a while Mr. S. called on his specialist, who said he had never known a case to have so greatly improved from the use of the drops he had given him to simply relieve the condition.

Again, later, another visit was made to the same specialist, who said he had never yet seen a case so completely cleared up from the use of these drops. The fact was, Mr. S. had not been using the drops at all since this Reflexology had been given to him.

Not caring to hurt the feelings of this specialist, nothing more was said, but Mr. S. was advised now by him to discontinue the use of the drops since the glaucoma had apparently disappeared.

EYES AND THEIR BLOOD SUPPLY

Remember this, where there is any trouble with the eyes caused by some bodily ailment, and you find the place between the toes very tender, it is certain you can help the condition by removing the crystals and replacing the normal circulation.

A tenderness at this point, as in any other place, means the eyes are being deprived of the proper blood supply, which means health and activity to any part of the body. You will notice rapid results from these treatments where there is a burning or itching condition of the eyes.

22

Ears

Now we find the ears too can be greatly benefited, but we will not try to tell you that all forms of deafness will respond to this treatment.

Deafness like blindness, can be caused by various conditions that may render it beyond all human power to restore. But from our past experience, we repeat again how this method has helped hundreds to a better degree of hearing.

Follow carefully the directions given for treating the eyes. The procedure is practically the same as far as the position for holding and grasping the foot is concerned. Only the reflex for the ears will be found between the third and fourth toes, while for the eyes we work principally between the second and third toes.

For the ears try also between the fourth and fifth toes, in other words hunt till you find a sore place. It is not advisable to follow any concrete rule as to locating these reflexes. It is impossible to tell in just what zone the trouble is that causes the deafness. With some it is one thing, and another something else entirely.

23

SURPRISING RESULTS OBTAINABLE

I shall not try to overestimate the amount of good that may be accomplished by this treatment, but I will say that you too, like myself, will be surprised many times at the astonishing results you will obtain where you might be expecting them the least. Especially if the deafness happens to be that which is caused by a catarrhal condition which is often the cause.

Enlarged Tonsils or Sore Throat

Now here comes a patient to you for help with a sore throat or enlarged tonsils. Where will you expect, on the foot, to find the reflex to the throat?

Since it is in the fleshy part of the big toe where we find the reflex to troubles in the head, naturally we will expect to find the throat reflexed at what we call the base of the big toe just at or a little above where it joins on to the foot as shown in Fig. 8.

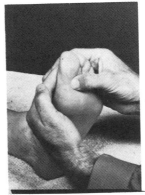

FIGURE 8

Position for Working the Reflex to the Throat.

Let me ask that you think a moment and picture in your mind that the throat is that part which connects the head to the body. Then just so will we find the tenderness reflecting to the throat in that part of the toe where it is connected to the foot. It will be necessary to use the first finger for the greater part of the work of this reflex, as you will have to reach around over the top of the toe on to that side between and facing the second toe. It will only require a little pressure here, not more than can be easily given with the first finger. The thumb may be used for working on the underside of this big toe.

Remember one thing, that the location of the tenderness around this big toe where you will work will depend on just what part or parts of the throat are mostly congested.

POSITION FOR REACHING THE REFLEX
TO THE THROAT

If the trouble or congestion in the throat is caused by an excessive amount of poison in the system, you may not get results till that condition has been cleared up, but if this congestion is not of too long standing as the result of a recent cold or sore throat, you will be surprised at what nature will do when she is given the proper amount and quality of blood with which to do her repair work.

You will be surprised how readily a stiff, lame neck will loosen up under this form of treatment around the big toe.

I have had a number of cases where it would seem as if the stiffness simply melted away and where they had come into the office not able to turn the head scarcely at all, they would go out almost as well as ever.

Sinus Trouble

This most annoying pain and trouble in the head is very perplexing to both the patient and the practitioner. It is claimed by some to be what was at one time known as catarrh of the head.

TEMPORARY RELIEF

The various forms of local treatment can afford some relief, but it is only temporary. They relieve the effect without doing anything to remove the cause.

Congestion, the keynote to all our aches and pains, whether it be a headache or a toeache, is the cause of our sinus trouble. If it is hard for you to believe it, try it out with this method and see for yourself if what I am telling you is true or not.

TENDERNESS IN TOES

Since this sinus trouble is in the head, we will find the reflex to this in the ten TOES. Where the congestion is severe and of long standing, it will be interesting to note the tenderness that will be found in, on, and around the toes. This will be observed especially as you press toward the base or root of each toe as shown in Fig. 4 and Fig. 9, from the outer and inner side on the ball of all ten toes.

The sides too, will be especially sensitive, and as you persistently continue this procedure, watch the results. The improvement will not be in a minute or over night. It will take time, the duration of which will depend entirely on the vitality and susceptibility to respond, and the length of time the condition has existed.

THE CAUSE AND EFFECT

If this sinus trouble is caused from a catarrhal condition in the system, the result of nature striving to overcome a hyperacidity in the body, we will do well to first try and remedy this condition; the cause of which you may have already found from the discovery of some tender reflex indicating what part or parts may be at fault.

NATURE DOES HER PART

Nature is constantly struggling to eliminate the waste matter of our body. The dead worn out body cells that are being constantly replaced by new ones, must be eliminated from our system in various ways.

One important avenue of escape for these poisons of the system is the pores of our skin. The mucous membrane in the head, nose, and sinus portion, being so much thinner at that particular place, gives nature a chance to discharge her surplus supply more easily through that channel. The result is, we have a discharge from the nose as nature succeeds in throwing it off. If instead, it becomes congested in the head, as in most cases of sinus trouble that have been known, then the trouble is more serious and painful, and you will wait longer for results.

But do not get discouraged, for as long as the slightest tenderness remains, you are still fighting with congestion.

27

Now where a condition of sinus trouble continues to exist, we know nature is still overburdened with this toxic acid mucous-forming condition and seeking constantly a form of elimination along the line of least resistance where the membrane lining is the thinnest.

EFFECTS OF A COLD

When you are overtaken by what is commonly known as a cold, remember this is nature's way of eliminating the toxic acid of the system. As a result we have an excessive amount of discharge from the nose and throat; because it is here where this acid can find its exit in the way of least resistance.

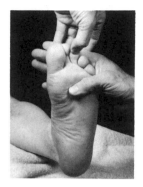

FIGURE 9

**Position for Working the Reflexes
to the Sinuses.**

The old method of soaking the feet in hot mustard water, taking a hot sweat bath, etc., all had its effect in relaxing and opening the pores of the body, helping nature in its process of elimination.

A PHYSICIAN'S METHOD

Our physician with his various remedies today for a cold, endeavors to bring about this same eliminating effect through the use of drugs as a more modern discovery. When people have completely recovered from a cold, note how much better they usually feel for the time being from this housecleaning method.

HAY FEVER

As late summer approaches you will often be asked if you can do anything to relieve or benefit a condition of hay fever with this form of Reflexology on the feet.

Without the slightest doubt, the same method we have just outlined for relief in cases of sinus trouble will also relieve one suffering from hay fever. In fact, I may safely say you will be surprised how quickly results will follow if you persistently work out all the tenderness you can find in, on and around all ten toes.

Glands

We find so many today suffering from various ailments, where the original cause can be traced to a gland deficiency. Remember every thought and emotion affects our glands and.every thought is either constructive or destructive. Our glands are health builders, each pouring out secretions, which if in harmony, health is the result. If any one of the seven principal glands of the body fail to function, our whole mechanism is out of order.

How necessary then that we remember the importance of right thinking. If we are filled with thoughts of fear, worry, anxiety, or grief, let us shift our mental gears and replace them with those of hope, cheer, courage and happiness. We must do it if we want to be one hundred percent well. If mentally depressed, try to associate with those who are optimistic, who are looking on the bright side of life. To be among those who have courage will help us to be more courageous and magnetic physically and mentally.

Our success in life depends on our ability to radiate a pleasing personality, which is wholly dependent on our thoughts and emotions and, how our glands are functioning, if in harmony or out of harmony.

We will now proceed to discuss the various forms of work allotted to the most important members of the gland family. We will first consider the Thyroid, and relate a few of the strange pranks for which this gland can be held responsible.

THE THYROID GLAND

When the Thyroid gland refuses to work, the baby no longer grows, but develops a vacant idiotic look. This gland acts somewhat as a spark generator and storage battery for the body. If we let our battery run down we get tired and gain weight rapidly, but if it becomes overcharged the

Thyroid secretion is excessive, the patient will be nervous, irritable, will lose weight and become emotionally unbalanced. Many times we find this condition responsible for our neurasthenics. It may be advisable to have a metabolism test taken to check up on the activity of this gland, but it has been proven that whatever the case may be, whether we must speed up or slow down the activity of this very important gland, we can usually bring about normal balance by this reflex on the foot leading to the Thyroid gland. Fig. 6. This will be found principally in the first and second zone on each foot at the base of the big toe, deeply seated, and must be reached by using the outside corner of the thumb as shown in Fig. 10.

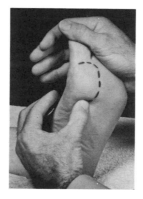

FIGURE 10
**Position for Working the Reflex Relative
to the Thyroid Gland**

In cases where there is a congestion leading away from the Thyroid toward the ear you will find it tender as you proceed with a deep pressure up between the first and second zones, between the big toe and the second toe. You will notice remarkable results from your work on this reflex. We have known them to gain as much as a pound a week where the gland was overactive and their weight far below normal.

EXOPHTHALMIC GOITRE

In this condition of goitre, the Thyroid gland enlarges, as in the case of simple goitre; the heart beat increases rapidly; the eyes bulge forward; the body becomes emaciated and very weak, and a nervous condition ensues. The growth itself may be scarcely noticeable, yet capable of doing a lot of mischief. Thus to work on the reflex to the Thyroid gland would help a condition of exophthalmic goitre.

We often find this condition has been brought about by a depressed mental attitude, grief or disappointment. No doubt you too, like myself, can recall many a case of this type which had its origin entirely around a thwarted love affair where a depressed desire had a definite effect on this particular gland interfering with its normal functioning.

It may take you longer to correct a case of this type unless you are successful in some way in changing the mental attitude or convincing the patient that to redirect the attention along some constructive line of endeavor is necessary for complete recovery.

THE PITUITARY GLAND

Some term the Pituitary as the master gland, for it has a powerful influence over the rhythm of the heart, beating time for the Adrenal and Thyroid glands in maintaining energy for the whole body. The Pituitary gland discharges certain hormones directly into the blood stream, playing an important part in our mode of living. It regulates our growth and governs, to a certain degree, the formation of sugar in our system.

A superactive Pituitary gland is responsible for the growth of our giants, while an inactive Pituitary is the cause of our dwarfs. If it goes haywire there is no telling what type of monstrosity may be produced.

Prof. Borgas, a surgeon of Rastov, Russia, capitalized in a dramatic way, on the growth-giving power of the Pituitary gland. From the brain of a young man, who an hour before had been killed in an automobile accident, Dr. Borgas cut out the Pituitary and grafted it into the stunted body of a fifteen year old girl, three feet tall. In six months she grew six inches.

Dr. James Hatton has had good results in reducing high blood pressure with carefully timed X-ray exposure to the back of the patient's head, and the kidneys, over the Pituitary and Adrenal regions.

If good results can be obtained by X-rays, then we know good results can be had by any method that will increase the circulation to that particular area. Suppose, as the result of congestion, this gland enlarges and becomes too big for the niche in which it rests, then a headache might follow. Not that all headaches are the result of an abnormal Pituitary, but this gland can do a lot of mischief.

A "STORY THE FEET DID TELL"

It may be interesting here to relate an experience I had one day last summer with an ex-champion wrestler who accompanied his wife to my office. Mr. G., with an exaggerated air of skepticism, stood by critically questioning Mrs. G. as to the necessity of her flinching as I worked the extremely tender reflexes of her feet. I endeavored to explain the cause of the tenderness at the nerve endings. Mr. G. confidently assured me I would find no tender place in his feet, saying, "I would like to meet the person who could make me flinch."

Since his appearance was that of one in perfect health I had no idea that we would be able to demonstrate to him the feeling of a tender reflex. After completing the Reflexology session on Mrs. G., she insisted that he should let me try the various reflexes of his feet. As I proceeded, I found no tenderness whatsoever until I reached that of the Pituitary gland as shown in Fig. 6 and Fig. 11. At this point he did not stop to flinch but nearly jumped off the table and cried out in no uncertain tones, that "it did hurt." To prove my findings I made sure the same tender spot existed in the center of each big toe and then I ventured to ask him if he had ever suffered from headaches.

In answering me he said it was impossible to describe the amount of suffering of the severity of the extreme headaches he had endured. It was almost unbelievable the amount of aspirin he had taken. And now comes the most unbelievable part of the story. After his third visit to my office this tenderness had completely worked out. While this took place almost a year ago he has had no return of his headaches. To verify this statement, I called on Mr. and Mrs. G. about a week ago. If any one feels inclined to doubt the truthfulness of this experience, their name and address will be cheerfully given.

As I have said before, if you will sincerely try Reflexology as directed in this book, you will affirm without fear of successful contradiction that congestion in the head as in any other part can often be relieved by this method of work on certain parts of the feet.

CONGESTION

The Pituitary is one of the smallest glands, being only the size of a pea and weighs about one-sixtieth of an ounce, and is situated in front of the medulla oblongata in the pituitary fossa of the sphenoidal bone.

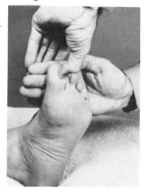

FIGURE 11

Position for Working the Reflex to the Pituitary Gland.

It has much to do with muscular strength and its removal would cause death. Its secretions are entirely internal, and are naturally taken into the system by absorption. Any means of stimulation to this gland, if properly given, will produce strength and health. I know of no better means of stimulating this gland than by this reflex method of ZONE THERAPY that we shall herein outline for your consideration. Note carefully the exact location as indicated in Fig. 6 and Fig. 11.

Since this gland is found resting in a groove at the base of the brain in a bony cradle just above the nasal cavity, we will find our reflex to this in the center of the big toe. You will invariably find this point tender, in cases of any glandular trouble, especially where there is a diabetic condition. It may be somewhat hard to find at first, but persistent pressure with the side of the thumb will be sure to locate it, and a few minutes attention given to working this gland at each treatment will often produce amazing results.

CASE RECORD

If anyone is inclined to doubt the effect that can be produced by deep pressure on the center of the big toe (the Pituitary reflex), read a case I here relate.

Mr. H., 63 years of age, had suffered with intense headaches for over five years dating back to a most serious operation when a brain tumor was removed. It was diagnosed as a cancerous type, and no hope was held out for his life, either during or after the operation. Beyond all expectation he survived and was able to be up and around his peaceful little home in the country, but never with any degree of comfort for he was annoyed with a constant headache during every waking hour, day or night. It was hard to even picture help for such a severe case caused by a most critical operation of this type.

The growth having been mostly on the right side of the head, led me to believe I would find the reflex to that part on the left foot, since certain nerve reflexes cross at the back of the neck. As I proceeded gently around the top of the big toe, on each side, etc., the tenderness was extreme. I continued working for about ten minutes, watching his expression intently so as to determine how deep and what pressure might be used without causing too much discomfort. I knew this tenderness was the result of congestion which must be released before there would be any degree of relief. Then, too, a condition of that kind would mean congestion possibly of the neck and shoulder on that side. So I proceeded to the reflex of the shoulder as shown in Fig. 2 and Fig. 20 and found this too, as tender as the reflex to the head. A little persistent work here at the base of the little toe, resulted in some immediate relief. After the third treatment Mr. H. turned to his wife and with tears of joy in his eyes exclaimed, "Mina, for the first time in five years, my headache is gone." The following summer found him again working in his garden.

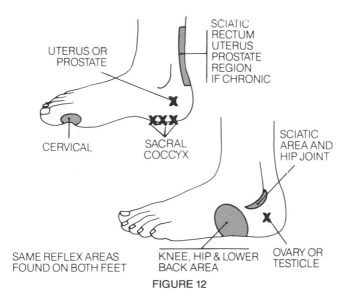

FIGURE 12

Another source of annoyance which added greatly to his discomfort, was that of an enlarged prostate gland, which not only increased his nervousness, but disturbed his rest at night by his being aroused six to eight times each night to urinate.

This meant work on the reflex to the prostate gland, which will be found midway between the ankle bone and edge of the heel as shown in Fig. 12.

With the heel of the left foot resting in the palm of your left hand, grasp the ankle with your right hand and try to locate this reflex with a firm rotary motion with the second and third fingers. Steadying your hand from the opposite side with the thumb and natural grasp of the ankle, will allow a free motion of the fingers to work on and around this particular part. It may take a few moments to locate the tender reflex, but remember where there is any abnormal condition of this gland there will be congestion with a formation of crystals at the nerve ending. This is what you are seeking to find and what you are going to break up, scattering the congestion and replacing the free normal circulation so nature can repair the sick, afflicted part. All she asks of us is to give her a chance.

Just as a person improperly fed and starving for the necessities of life would be incapable of working proficiently, so it is with any portion of our body. If we cut off any part of the circulation with calcium or crystalline deposits, we deplete the functioning of those particular glands and their associate members.

The Pancreas

SHAPE AND LOCATION

The Pancreas is a compound racemose gland of pyramidal shape about six to eight inches long, one and a half inches wide and one inch thick. It is situated transversely across the posterior wall of the abdomen, behind the stomach and in front of the second lumbar vertebra.

The Pancreatic duct extends the whole length of the gland and opens into the descending part of the duodenum to the inner side, with the common bile duct. As a ductless gland this capable organ secretes from its insular cells, insulin, which acts as a draft to a furnace in burning up the excessive sugar in the system.

While the liver and Pancreas secrete differently, the secretions of both are affected in diabetes. It is the function of the Pancreas to secrete pancreatic juice and also a fluid of great digestive power known as insulin which burns up or consumes any excessive sugar that might be in the blood stream as the result of a torpid liver.

It is the work of the liver to secrete bile, but if it fails to do this normally, abnormal secretions take place and an oversupply of sugar is manufactured in the liver. Then in the face of this if we find a depleted Pancreas unable to send out this important insulin, as a draft to the furnace in burning it up, the blood stream becomes overloaded with sugar and that spills over into the urine, and overburdens the kidneys, too, in throwing it off.

Diabetes

What you are interested in now will be to know if anything can be done to help this Pancreas, since it is failing to perform its duty as shown by the presence of sugar in the urine. You will be sure to find its reflex tender, indicating the presence of crystals in the nerve endings. Then as you proceed working this reflex according to the location outlined in Fig. 13, you will be breaking up these deposits, supplying this gland with a better blood supply which will in time wake it up to a better performance of its duty.

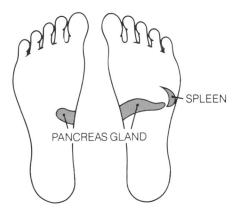

SPLEEN

PANCREAS GLAND

FIGURE 13

I have had astonishing results with Refexology in cases of Diabetes but it takes time and patience.

As in every ailment, we find some who respond more readily than others; so do not get discouraged. It has completely cleared up the condition for many.

INSULIN NOT A CURE

If the urine is being tested carefully during this time, it will be interesting to note the increase of sugar showing in the tests the day following your work on this reflex.

The increase in circulation evidently stimulates the liver to throw off more of its excessive load of sugar.

If insulin is being used, by all means keep it up until the tests improve sufficiently to warrant a gradual decrease. If under the care of a physician, he will order the amount to be cut down as the tests improve, for he will be as anxious as you are to see the units of insulin decreased. Insulin is not a cure, but acts only as a crutch to bolster up and supply that which is deficient in the system. The same as if you have a broken limb, the crutch is needed only until that which has been injured is again able to perform its duty.

Asthma and the Adrenal Glands

Asthma, we all know, is a very disagreeable ailment. It is not considered particularly dangerous, but it can cause a lot of discomfort, and may continue with a devastating effect on the system over a period of years and almost a lifetime in some extreme cases. It is considered a condition where the phlegm hardens in the bronchial tubes.

Since the cause seems to vary in different individuals, it is impossible to expect relief in every case from any one method or form of treatment. We all know that extreme attacks are usually relieved by the use of adrenalin either by hypodermic injection or inhalation of the spray. Would it not seem possible then if we could increase the supply of adrenalin in the system, we might in most cases bring about relief?

LOCATION OF THE ADRENAL GLANDS

We will first call to mind the location of these very important glands, as they sit like little caps atop each kidney, so closely connected with and related to the kidneys that it would be impossible to determine a difference between the reflex to the kidneys and that of the Adrenal glands.

Nevertheless let us remember that we cannot stimulate circulation to one without helping the other; and since it is so important to one suffering from asthma to have a sufficient supply of adrenalin secretion, let us concentrate on doing all in our power to stimulate a better action on these important glands.

NOTHING MORE PRECIOUS

There is nothing more precious to the well-being of an individual than a good pair of Adrenal glands. It is the adrenalin secretion that stimulates the action of the heart.

The emotion of fear plays an important part on these adrenalin secretions. Strength is hidden within these glands, which is brought into effect in times of immediate danger. It is the secretion from a good pair of Adrenal glands that gives us courage and strength to successfully cope with an emergency in life. The strength and success of our great athletes and prize fighters all depend on the condition and activity of their Adrenal glands.

The same important secretion governs the amount of vitality and resistance built up in our body to fight and resist disease. Then allow me to say we can make no mistake in doing anything that will increase the circulation and stimulate the secretions of such an important pair of glands.

I have never yet found a case of asthma where the reflexes to these glands were not tender. Asthma, like any other malady, will not be found in a perfectly healthy body where every gland and organ is functioning in perfect harmony. Thus, many a case of asthma will respond readily to this method when used on the reflex to the Adrenal glands. Fig. 6. It may take a while in some cases where the difficulty has existed for many years. But time and a little persistent effort on your part will conquer many a seeming impossibility.

Do Nerves Affect
Skin Action?

It is allotted to our skin to throw off and send out three pints of poison a day. It is said if this were to be injected back into the blood stream we would die in three days of blood poisoning.

Now suppose we are all tightened up worrying over something that tenses and tightens all the pores of the body so that we fail to throw off this allotted portion of poison. We are then increasing the burden of the kidneys and heart which have so much to do with the elimination of the poisons of the body.

ECZEMA

This I give here as a thought to remember in any case of skin eruption, especially eczema. First see if the kidney action is interfered with by a formation of crystalline deposits in the nerve endings—see if they might be in this way hindered in doing their important part of eliminating the uric acid from the system, thus placing an extra burden on the pores of the skin.

42

The Heart

A GREAT PUMPING STATION

Our heart, our blood and its circulation, are most important factors of our being. It is said that 156 pounds per hour of this precious life giving fluid pass through this great pumping station called the heart, on its round to supply the body with nourishing material.

In the Dresden Hygiene Exposition it was shown that 24 quarts of blood pass through the circulatory system in three minutes. In twenty-four hours the heart does enough work to lift three men to the top of a building 44 feet high. Is it any wonder this great organ would grow weary at times?

SIZE, WEIGHT, ETC.

The heart is a hollow muscular organ of a conical form, placed between the lungs and enclosed in the cavity of the pericardium, obliquely in the chest. The broad attached end or base, is directed upwards to the right and corresponds to the interval between the fifth and eighth dorsal vertebrae. The apex is directed forwards and to the left and corresponds to the interspace between the cartilages of the fifth and sixth ribs.

The heart in an adult measures about five inches in length, three and a half inches in breadth, and two and a half inches in thickness. The prevalent weight in the male varies from ten to twelve ounces in proportion to the size of the body.

LOCATING THE REFLEX TO THE HEART

We find the heart and the muscles surrounding it and governing its activity will be reflexed strongly in the left foot and principally in the second, third and fourth zones. Its being embedded deep in the body will necessitate considerable pressure in some cases.

Now with the heel of the left foot resting on the palm of your left hand, use your right thumb; try to locate the reflex at the base of the third and fourth toes as shown in Fig. 14 and Fig. 3.

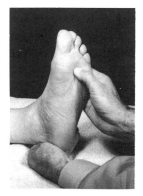

FIGURE 14
**Position for Working the Reflex
to the Heart.**

I suggest you use the inside corner of the thumb for this. It may require a little time and considerable pressure to find the reflex not knowing the exact location of the trouble, whether it be with or around the heart. But any tenderness will be evidence of congestion, and you will have no difficulty in convincing the patient that something is not quite normal, as evident from the tenderness discovered by your pressure on the reflex.

EFFECTS OF CONGESTION

If the slightest congestion takes place among the arteries and veins surrounding the heart and this condition remains long enough, what usually happens — why, we soon hear of heart attacks.

CONGESTION FORMS CLOTS

Congestion forms clots, and these disturb the vascular action of the heart, called embolus (blood clot in the blood vessels). To call a condition of this kind, "heart disease," is a misnomer. It is like blaming the engine for the poor performance of our automobile, when actually the trouble is caused by an obstruction in the gasoline line robbing it of the necessary amount of gas needed for the proper functioning of the motor.

Palpitation may be caused solely from indigestion. As the stomach, filling with gases formed from undigested food, distends and presses against the diaphragm, it appears to disturb the heart.

AS COMPARED TO A WATCH

Remember the network of muscles constituting the heart and the various valves and intricate parts that go to make up this most important organ. When studying the anatomy of the heart, it always reminds me of a watch, with so many wheels and parts to get out of order.

By this time we can readily understand how undue nerve tension, congestion, etc., in and around the heart, would tend to slow up the action, and finally cause it to stop. Like dust in the delicate wheels of a watch, only sometimes we can restore a watch to action by flushing it with some form of fluid.

But the heart can never be restored when once it has ceased to beat. It is before it stops that it must be flushed with the proper blood supply, which you will be able to give it by freeing these nerve endings of all acid or calcium deposits where there is a tender reflex. Suppose you find no tenderness in this region; then you know the trouble must be something other than of the heart itself. In many cases of heart trouble, results may follow quickly, for so many times, as we have explained, you will find what has been mistaken for heart trouble is only some nerve tension or some tightened muscle, which, when relaxed, will restore the heart again to its normal action.

Let me suggest that your work for the heart be given rather easy at first. When you find the tender place, work on it for two or three contacts, then let that place rest, while you work some other parts, then return to it again. Do this several times alternating.

AN UNUSUAL CASE

I will relate one experience I had two years ago. The lady, a personal friend of mine, was living in the country some distance away.

I knew she had been troubled with heart attacks for several years, and it was on this account she had been obliged to retire to the quietude of a country home. When I became acquainted with the work I could do for the heart with this reflex method, I wrote immediately for her to come, which she readily did. And at once I found the tender reflex, located as I have outlined it in Fig. 14.

She pleaded for mercy, and insisted I was using something sharp, as a piece of glass, instead of the end of my thumb.

Finally she cried out, "Stop a minute," and said to me, "What have you done?"

I hestitated and said laughingly, "Why nothing."

She said, "Oh, yes you have," and then she went on to explain that it had felt as if a streak of lightning had flashed from her foot to her heart, followed by the sensation as if some stimulant had been administered.

I did no more at that time, but left nature to do her part.

Now to all appearances I had opened up some new channel, doing something to the circulation. For two days following she experienced a feeling of exhaustion, "just all in," as she described it, then she began to pick up. After a few more treatments the soreness had disappeared, but never again did she feel the streak of lightning effect. She gained rapidly in strength and was able to work and do things she had been denied the privilege of doing for several years, and since that time she has been able to do her work as well as anyone.

She has never had another similar heart attack.

A PHYSICIAN'S ADVICE

While relating this incident one day to a noted heart specialist, I asked Dr. B. to tell me what, in his opinion, had caused the sensation of a streak of lightning to shoot from her foot to her heart, while I was working that particular reflex. His reply was this. Pointing his finger at me, he said, "You obtained results, didn't you? Then that is all that counts. Just keep it up."

That is exactly what I intend to do whenever I am given the chance. That is why I am trying to pass this on to you that others too may be helped in the same way, and to the same extent this friend of mine has been.

ANGINA PECTORIS

I have had a number of cases of angina pectoris respond very readily to these reflex treatments. Let me say if the pain extends up toward the shoulder and neck, work up toward the root of the fourth and fifth toes. Keep trying till you find the tenderness, then set to and work it out. I cannot lay down any stereotyped rule for you to follow, but you must work on the foot according to the location of the pain around the heart. If the pain extends down toward the arm, work around the base of the little toe, as pointed out and directed for trouble in the shoulder.

Since it is certain no harm can be done by working on a reflex, there is no need to hesitate, but set out and do all the good that can be accomplished.

With a short plump person we will find everything more compact, with one organ lying back of another, etc. and closer together than those of the taller more slender person.

The Gall Bladder

The gall bladder is a pear-shaped fibro muscular receptacle for the bile. Its length is from three to four inches, and its breadth about one inch. Its capacity is from eight to twelve fluid-drams and it is lined with mucous membranes. It is lodged in a fossa on the under surface of the right lobe of the liver.

GALL STONES

This we find to be a very painful trouble caused by the bile which instead of passing through the common bile duct into the duodenum, coagulates itself into hardened masses called gall stones. You can see what an important part is played here, where anything might exist causing or increasing any form of congestion.

CASE RECORD

You will be interested to hear about one particular case. Mrs. O. had been in poor health for some time. Finally it was considered necessary for her to undergo a major operation. While she was on the operating table, the doctor discovered a large stone in the gall bladder, which they considered dangerous to remove at that time because it would have kept her under an anesthetic too long. She was told she would have to return to the hospital as soon as her recovery would permit and have this stone removed.

In the meanwhile she came to me. This stone was troubling her frequently, causing severe pain attacks so that she was unable to move her arms at times. She could never reach down to pick anything up off the floor with the right arm.

I found the reflex to this sick gall bladder very tender, and believe it or not, it took only a few treatments to work out the congestion of this reflex and the pain disappeared. Fig. 15 and Fig. 16.

Now she can use her arm as well as ever; can reach up or down without the slightest discomfort, and has had no return of the pain attacks.

Mrs. O. and I often speak of this stone the doctor discovered, and we wonder what has become of it. Evidently it must have dissolved or the treatment relaxed the gall duct sufficiently so that it passed off without her knowing it.

Another case interesting to mention. Mrs. J. had experienced a number of acute gall bladder attacks, each one seemingly more severe than the one before. She could picture nothing but an operation for relief. As in all such cases, I found the reflex to the gall bladder most tender. The day following her first treatment, in the exact location of the pain center, she had a most peculiar sensation which she described as feeling like worms crawling. By stretching her body in various ways the sensation would cease for a few minutes and then return. The next day it let up gradually, and finally disappeared. This happened a year ago and Mrs. J. has had no return of the pain attacks.

If congestion causes these stones to form in the beginning there is no telling what nature will do if we give her chance, by relieving this congestion, which is sure to take place when the tenderness has been thoroughly worked out.

The Liver

The Liver is the largest gland in the body. It is located in the right side of the body and weighs about three pounds in a full grown person. Its transverse diameter is about eleven inches, its anterior posterior about eight, and its greatest vertical, five to seven inches.

It is rightly named the "King of the Glands." It is the largest organ in the body, and has within it at all times, about one-quarter of all the blood in the body circulating through it.

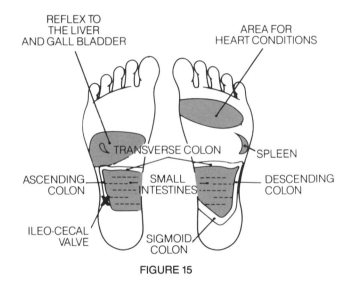

REFLEX TO
THE LIVER
AND GALL BLADDER

AREA FOR
HEART CONDITIONS

TRANSVERSE COLON

SPLEEN

ASCENDING
COLON

SMALL
INTESTINES

DESCENDING
COLON

ILEO-CECAL
VALVE

SIGMOID
COLON

FIGURE 15

DIFFERENT TASKS

The Liver must perform many tasks. It manufactures bile to digest fats and prevent constipation; it is a natural antiseptic and purgative; and it helps to supply some of the substances for blood making. The liver stores up sugar within itself for future uses. It is a great filter, taking the excessive and venomous matter and waste tissues of the body and secreting and forming its own weight normally, or about two pints of bile per day. This goes into the intestines to lubricate and prevent constipation.

How necessary it is that this very important organ should function correctly, which is only possible when it receives the proper circulation.

SLUGGISH LIVER

When the liver is sluggish and fails to do its work efficiently, we must stimulate the circulation to the muscular tissues controlling the liver and the nerves which cause it to operate.

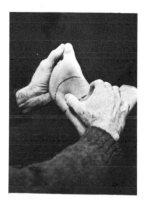

FIGURE 16
**Position for Working the Reflex
to the Liver.**

When we find in the foot a tenderness in the region of the reflex to the liver as shown in Fig. 15 and Fig. 16, we know the liver is sluggish and failing to function properly.

We also know it lacks the proper circulation and muscular action necessary to keep sending the blood to the particular extremities of the feet with sufficient force to prevent a formation of crystals responsible for this tenderness in these nerve endings, which gradually increases, continuing to impede the normal circulation.

We all admit that as this condition continues over a period of days, weeks, months, and even years, we weaken the normal functions of this great important gland, and the results may be jaundice, diabetes, gall stones, atrophy, sclerosis, constipation, etc. Now as we continue working with a firm creeping pressure, deep into the sensitive reflex where these crystals are formed, we are able to dissolve them, lessening the obstruction so that the natural circulation can be restored. From the striking reactions we have obtained, there is no doubt of the powerful results obtainable from this Method of Reflexology.

Case Record

I will here mention the reaction in the case of Mrs. H., who had been confined to an invalid chair for six years, as the result of a severe back injury.

Being unable to exercise properly, the liver had become dormant, and even the slightest pressure caused severe pain over this region of the foot. After the third treatment this sluggish liver had received sufficient blood supply to increase its activity, and Mrs. H. had sixteen bowel movements in twenty-four hours.

EFFECTS DISCERNIBLE

You will find in every case, where a sluggish liver is involved, or any ailment resulting from this condition, that the reaction will be a tired, lifeless feeling; for nature is now struggling to combat the excessive amount of poison being eliminated from the liver during this house cleaning period. The stools at this time may be black, green, yellow or heavy mucus.

The location pointed out in these various illustrations will give you as best we can, the approximate location for a working basis. For instance, where the liver is greatly enlarged, we will find a larger portion of the foot involved. The reflex to a badly prolapsed colon will also show in a little lower position on the foot.

Not long ago I was called to the bedside of Mr. K., age seventy-one years, who had been confined to his bed for three weeks. Several doctors had been in attendance, all expressing their opinion that Mr. K. had a very bad heart, and his weight being over three hundred pounds, none offered any hope of recovery. He had often, of late, become delirious, telling his children he had only a few more days to live.

I gave a very light treatment the first time, finding the reflex to the liver most tender. I explained the kind of reaction to expect when the circulation to that sick sluggish liver would be increased and sure enough, while the first treatment relaxed his nerves and made it possible for him to sleep without the aid of sleeping powders, the second treatment given three days later had the opposite effect.

For about twenty-four hours Mr. K. was restless, delirious, and manifesting in various ways that the increased circulation, produced by this work over the reflex area on the foot leading to the liver, had released congestion, making it necessary for nature to put forth an extra effort to eliminate the excess poison.

53

After the third treatment given three days later, Mr. K. felt a great deal better and each treatment thereafter produced a marked improvement till he was soon up and around again.

DO NOT TREAT TOO OFTEN

If the reaction is severe, do not give another treatment too soon. Let a few days elapse to give nature a chance to adjust itself to the increased circulation.

VARICOSE VEINS

It is claimed by some that where there is a condition of varicose veins, we find trouble with the liver. Believe this or not, let me say when you have learned this method you will never be afraid of any case of varicose veins. For with the proper circulation, that congestion will disappear; just so with cramps or pains of any kind in the limbs.

The Back

How many people we find today who ask for some way or method of relief for a lame back.

A little study of the chart, Fig. 1, and you will acquaint yourself with the location of the zones in reference to the back.

The whole spinal column, being in the exact center of the body where the zones divide, will give us the reflex for the spine in the first zone of each foot, which will cover the entire area of the inner side of the foot lengthwise from the toe to the heel.

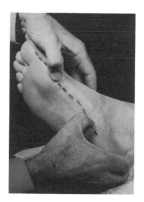

FIGURE 17
**Position for Working the Reflex
to the Back.**

55

The big toe represents that of the head; the center of the foot, the center of the back or waistline of the body; the lower part of the foot or inner part down toward the heel, the lower part of the back. See Fig. 5.

Keep this picture in your mind and it will be no trouble to find the exact location of the trouble or weakness in the back from the location of the tenderness on the inner side of the foot.

IMPINGED NERVES

The same method outlined in this book for helping other parts of the body will hold good here too. Remember every part of our body receives its nerve supply from some part of the spine, and a big majority of our ailments today can be traced to some misplacement or impinged nerve tightening the muscles of some part holding it that way with this abnormal tension.

Now since we can prove beyond a mistake or doubt that this method of working on the reflexes has a definite relaxing effect, just what is going to take place as you continue to work on the reflex to the spine if it is in any way out of alignment? What will happen is this: as you relax the tension in the spinal cord your muscles will cease to contract and in the natural ways and walks of life the vertebra that was once out of alignment will often replace itself to the natural position, supplying those parts again with the proper circulation.

Congestion will take wings and fly away. The worn out depleted body cells of that part affected from this impingement will be replaced by new ones from the fresh supply of blood received now from a more perfect source of circulation.

PURE BLOOD

If you cut off any part of the blood supply to any portion of the body, you are increasing the congestion and slowing down the circulation, when circulation is the most important factor to a pure life-giving blood stream.

You are familiar with the difference between a still pool of water and a flowing stream; while the water of one becomes foul and stagnant, the other purifies itself through the oxygen in the air. Our blood purifies itself in proportion to the oxygen it picks up on its way as it passes through the lungs.

Before leaving this subject on what to do for any lameness of the back, let me relate a case record quite unusual.

CASE RECORD

Ten years ago Mrs. S. met with an automobile accident when she was thrown under the front of a truck. Lying on her back she reached forward and in some way, no one knows how, she pulled herself out from under it. In doing so she severely hurt her back. The injury was most severely deep under each shoulder blade. She soon recovered from the other minor injuries she sustained, but this pain in her back never did cease. She persistently tried every method suggested but nothing afforded relief.

Very skeptically she came to me. She was advised by a friend who came with her not to tell me where or in what part of her back the trouble existed, but to see if I could locate it from her feet. As soon as I proceeded (beginning at the top under the big toe) with this heavy pressure and began to work down, I soon reached the reflex to that part under the shoulder blades—at this point she flinched. I then knew I had found the trouble; but before asking her, I made sure there were no other tender reflexes.

Checking it carefully and finding it the same on the other foot, somewhat worse on the left than the right, I ventured to ask if her trouble might not be directly under the shoulder blades, in very deep about three to four inches from the center of the spine and worse on the left than the right side. She verified this as being exactly correct.

After a very few treatments, the trouble disappeared. There was a vivid reaction. The first night it ached severely, but the second and third treatments given every third day gradually began to bring relief till it finally disappeared entirely. She could then do her housework and use a broom to sweep for the first time since the accident.

Disorders of the Kidneys

The kidneys are involved in all forms of Bright's Disease, and usually in diabetic troubles.

The kidneys may be enlarged or they may be atrophied, or decreased below the normal size. They may be loosened or floated somewhat from their normal position. They may secrete either too much or not enough urine. As we have said before, any condition that is abnormal will interfere with the health of the individual. If the muscular action becomes insufficient to keep the nerve endings free from all crystalline deposits, these important organs of elimination will fail to function properly.

Now since circulation is responsible for all bodily and mental functions, and the kidneys being the eliminators of poisons from the system, the logical conclusion is that, if we can do anything to increase the circulation, we will enable the kidneys to a greater efficiency in carrying off the toxins or poisons of the system.

In dropsy it is most important to secure good and full kidney action which will at once reduce the swollen and puffed condition of the body. Where a condition of this kind exists you will be amazed at the results which can be obtained by this method on the reflexes to the kidneys.

Remember we have two kidneys, one on the right side of the body and one on the left. Thus, we find the reflex to the right kidney in the right foot; the left kidney in the left foot, as shown in Fig. 5 and Fig. 19.

Since a number of ailments may result from a pair of lazy kidneys, let me say you will be surprised at how often you will find these reflexes tender. You will have astonishing results many times, even from the first treatment.

Let me warn you again, if you have a severe case of kidney trouble, do not overdo the work or treat too often, for this form of treatment will have a powerful effect on the kidneys. It will take nature just so long, even with the renewed amount of circulation, to replace the old diseased kidney cells with new ones capable of sufficiently eliminating the uric acid from the system.

So just have a little patience—15 minutes every third or fourth day is often enough in most cases. For an extreme case I would suggest only once a week at first, until nature can readjust itself.

LUMBAGO

One of the most painful conditions that so often follows where the kidneys fail to do their part in eliminating the uric acid from the system is what we know as lumbago or a catch in the back.

The latest method for relief in cases of this kind is to have the patient go to bed and lie on a board for a week or two. We can imagine how this would feel when the pain is simply excruciating at even the slightest move.

But, if one is not familiar with this work on the feet, they can only hope for relief in any way suggested by the physician.

59

A Case Record

To relate one of my experiences in this line will explain more fully what can really be accomplished with this method of Reflexology.

Mrs. H., apparently feeling as well as usual, was mopping her kitchen floor. As she finished, she reached over to pick up the pail and was instantly seized with this extremely painful catch in her back. She was unable to move and fell to the floor. Being alone in the house, it was nearly an hour before anyone arrived to help her up. It was impossible to get her undressed and into bed until the physician arrived to administer a sedative hypodermic injection.

Since I was out of town at the time, it was not until the following day that I could see her. She had spent a terrible night trying to lie on the ironing board. When I arrived I had to reach over the foot of the bed to work on her feet as it was impossible at first to move her feet over the edge of the bed, as we usually do when treating a patient in bed.

I first took the right foot in my left hand and with my right thumb I began to work the reflex to the lower part of the back as shown in Fig. 17 and 3. It was extremely tender and Mrs. H. insisted she could feel the effect of it right then in the lower end of her spine where we knew the trouble existed. I worked first on one foot then the other till the tenderness finally disappeared. By this time she could move around without the pain. For the first time since seized with this attack, she was able to move with but little pain and when I was ready to leave she got up and putting on her robe and slippers, walked into the living room. While she was still somewhat weak and shaky from the pain she had endured, the catch no longer existed and she was soon doing her work again as usual.

It is not any wonder that Mr. H. has such a great deal of faith in what can be accomplished through working the reflexes of the feet; for two years ago she was suffering with diabetes, living on the strictest diet, and weighing 96 pounds when she first came to me. Her twin sister had just passed away with this same dread disease.

I shall not try to tell you how soon she began to improve for not everyone will be able to respond so readily but, now for two years, Mrs. H. has been able to eat everything without the slightest trace of sugar showing in her urine; and today weighs 146 pounds.

If anyone is inclined to doubt this story in any way, she will be glad to have me give them her name and address so she can verify what I have said.

This is only one of a number of cases I have had where

a catch can be immediately relieved by thoroughly working the reflex to the lower lumbar region of the spine.

A little experience will help you to find the approximate location. As I have said before, if you find a tender spot, it means congestion and something which must be worked out before your patient will be one hundred percent well.

As you become accustomed to this work, if your thumbs are at all sensitive, many times it will be possible for you to feel a gritty substance as you apply the firm slow creeping movement with the ball of your thumb. Not in every case will you be able to feel these crystalline deposits, but I find more often with those where the muscles are firm it requires considerable pressure to find the reflexes. At least you will feel a difference at the point where the reflex is most tender. Sometimes it is in the form of a thick, more solid substance which will gradually disappear as your work continues.

Paralysis

From this point let us consider the fate of one suffering from the effects of a stroke of apoplexy, the cause of which we all know to be that of a hemorrhage somewhere in the brain, usually on just one side, causing a partial or wholly paralyzed condition on the opposite side of the body to that of the head where the hemorrhage occurred.

CLOT CAUSING PRESSURE

Now consider the condition the patient is in. This tiny clot caused from the hemmorhage is causing an undue pressure on that part of the brain which governs the motor action of that half of the body which is paralyzed. The brain is unable to send a command through the delicate nerve setup of our body and thus it remains lifeless.

Whether or not the condition will improve depends on how severe the hemorrhage has been, which we know too well all happens very suddenly and without any warning. Nevertheless, there may be a marked improvement if nature has endowed the individual with the necessary vitality to partially absorb this clot.

As the absorption of this clot takes place, it will permit a better message transference to go through from the brain to that part, the affected side, without being so heavily clouded with static. This seems to somewhat illustrate the condition that takes place.

WILL REFLEXOLOGY HELP?

Now before we say whether this REFLEXOLOGY method may be of any benefit to such a case, let us check back and see why this hemorrhage took place.

There was a real cause, and that cause we know is generally found to be high blood pressure. Let us see if the kidneys, liver, intestines, etc. are doing their part proficiently. Unless some injury might have taken place, we know there was a cause, a primary condition responsible for this high blood pressure. This condition will still be evident after the shock, so with the information we have been giving you as to the location of the reflexes, and the stories they tell of congestion and trouble, no doubt you will soon place your finger on the keynote to the whole difficulty.

CAUSE AND EFFECT

Whatever is wrong, as the location of the tenderness will determine, set out to correct it before expecting any great improvement. Try to find and remove the cause of the high blood pressure. Then see what you can do to help the circulation of the blood to dissolve this clot as much as possible.

By doing this, you will help remove the static, thereby getting a better, a more distinct message through to the various parts of the afflicted side. We never move a finger or a toe without a message being sent through to that part from the brain guiding and directing that move, however slight it may be.

63

REFLEX IN THE TOES

From what has already been said regarding the various locations of the zones and reflexes, you will readily assume that the reflex to any part of the brain will be found in the big toes. Remember some of the nerves cross at the back of the neck, so where we find the left side of the body paralyzed we may look for the reflex to this in the big toe on the right foot. Then work the big toe on the opposite side of the body to that which is afflicted. See if any part of this toe is tender, if so work it out. By doing this you are increasing the circulation to the location of the clot in the brain, helping nature in its work of absorption. It is also advisable to work both big toes, which will be a benefit to the whole head.

BENEFIT FROM REFLEXOLOGY

One case I worked on, the whole big toe became black and blue following the treatment, and he reported feeling better by far the following day than he had at any time since his second shock a year ago. He did then recall the same toe being black and blue especially around the nail at the time of his stroke. Why it was then, and why it should be again now that I was working on it, stands out with a big question mark for you to find the answer. It was not the pressure I used that caused it either, that I know.

Let me say that the more you study along this line and begin to work on these principles for yourself, you will become more convinced every day that what I am telling you is true, and that there is still a vast field for discovery in FOOT REFLEXOLOGY.

Sciatica

The great sciatic nerve supplies nearly the whole of the integument of the leg, the muscles of the back of the thigh, and of the leg and foot. It is the largest nerve cord in the body, measuring three quarters of an inch in breadth, and is the continuation of the lower part of the sacral plexus. It passes out of the pelvis through the great sacrasciatic foramen. It descends along the back part of the thigh to about its lower third, where it divides into two large branches, the internal and external popliteal nerves. If you will review your study of anatomy and examine carefully a diagram showing the posterior view of the nerves of the lower extremity, you will readily understand why this nerve can be reached through our work on the feet and on the inner side of the ankle, above and back of the ankle bone where the nerve lies nearest the surface.

Should the pressure of your thumb be too severe, try using the tip of the third finger, holding the ankle firmly in the palm of the same hand and the heel steadied with a firm grasp of the other hand. In a severe case of sciatica, where the inflammation has been of long standing, do not be surprised if the first few treatments bring tears to the eyes of your patient. To prevent this if possible, watch carefully the expression, so as to quickly let up as soon as you feel you have gone the limit of what the patient can stand. Here you must use care and let the pressure be gradual, and steadily increase as the pain subsides.

WHAT CAUSES SCIATICA?

Sciatica is generally accepted as the result of some misplacement along the lumbar region. But we find, too, there can be other causes for this painful malady, such as an enlargement of the prostate gland or injury to some other part of the body affecting the sciatic nerve.

It was a case of this type I had the pleasure of relieving a short time ago. Mr. P., a man about 55 years of age, came to me with but little faith in his heart that I would be able to help his case with my method of work on his feet. For eight years he had suffered untold agony. He had been confined to his bed for days and weeks at a time, and he had spent a small fortune as you can imagine any one would do in such a painful condition, visiting the very best and most reputable physicians the medical or drugless profession had to offer. The question remained, would I be able to locate, in my simple way, the cause and relief for this exceptionally stubborn case? I decided it could be no misplacement in the lumbar region as that would have been corrected long ago. I reasoned that the cause in this case was different. I would be sure to find a formation of crystals in that great nerve ending somewhere in the foot and leg that had failed to respond to any other form of treatment. As I proceeded with the end of my thumb, in a slow, creeping motion on that part of the foot as shown in Fig. 17, reflex for the lower lumbar region, there was no longer a question as to the congestion in the lumbar area. I proceeded up the inside and outside of the ankle, above and back of the ankle bone, till I found more and more of these crystals. Even the slightest pressure in these regions caused intense pain.

After about twenty minutes work on the affected side and ten minutes working alternately on the other foot, which was also somewhat tender, Mr. P. arose and in walking around could immediately feel some relief. After several treatments given every third day, there was a decided improvement, especially the day following each treatment. As I became impatient for somewhat quicker results, Mr. P. would constantly remind me that his was a case of eight years standing, and that I was already doing more for him than anyone else had done.

One evening, having a little spare time after the treatment, I set out to question Mr. P. to see if I might determine the cause. Calling to mind the rules of ZONE THERAPY, and the reflex relation of one part of the body to the other as taught by Dr. Fitzgerald, I inquired if he might at any time in the past have injured his shoulder, or arm on that afflicted side. This he heartily confirmed by showing me how impossible it was to raise that arm properly, it having been broken and improperly set, then rebroken several times, endeavoring to remedy the first injury. This had happened four or five years before the sciatic trouble had set in. Now the question arises: Could these injured nerves in the shoulder have any reflex action in the hip that could lessen the normal circulation of the great sciatic nerve, or will we say cause a short circuit in some way? We leave you to guess. We do know something had certainly impeded the circulation, burning off the insulation to cause so much inflammation and discomfort.

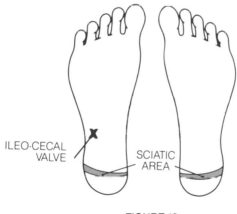

ILEO-CECAL VALVE

SCIATIC AREA

FIGURE 18

The extreme tenderness in that foot meant an exaggerated formation of crystals that had gradually been increasing as the trouble continued.

Let the cause be what it may, I found certain parts of the shoulder very tender, which I thoroughly worked. Then to help this I returned to the reflex in the foot leading to the shoulder as shown in Fig. 20 and Fig. 21 and Fig. 22, which was also very tender. With all these forces brought to bear, it was only a reasonable time till Mr. P. was entirely free from every particle of pain. It is my candid belief that his whole trouble had its origin in that injury to his shoulder.

When inflammation of this great sciatic nerve exists, we can readily understand why it would be a most painful and soul-racking disease. But it can be easily relieved by the simple method we herein set forth, if accompanied with persistent effort and a little patience, which is the only way to accomplish anything worth while.

Bursitis

While we are calling your attention to the location on the foot having a reflex action on the shoulder, let me tell you what can be done for many a lame aching shoulder, that may have refused to respond to other forms of treatment.

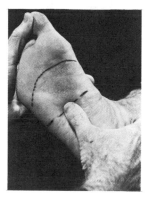

FIGURE 19

**Position for Working the Reflex
to the Kidneys.**

I recall a case of bursitis. The young lady, a telephone operator, had been disabled for nearly a year. It was impossible to raise the arm more than a few inches from her body. She was discouraged, for nothing yet had offered any relief. Many forms of heat and electricity had been applied, which only increased the pain.

Now we know in any case of bursitis we are handling inflammation of the bursa, and until this inflammation has subsided, it is not advisable to work directly over the afflicted part. Then let us concentrate our efforts on the reflex to this shoulder as pointed out in Fig. 20.

You will find as we shall call it the root of the little toe representing that of the shoulder, and as you press firmly in and around that area you will find some extremely tender spot which can be worked out in time, having a definite effect on the afflicted shoulder without any direct contact with the shoulder itself.

CAUSES OF BURSITIS

In a case of this kind we must always look for what might be the cause of bursitis, neuritis, rheumatism, or such kindred ailments. See if the kidneys are not lazy and refusing to throw off the uric acid sufficiently to prevent an acid condition of the blood, as was definitely the cause of the case I just mentioned. This young lady was being treated for Bright's Disease at the time she came to my office. As I proceeded to work the reflex to the kidneys, which was extremely sensitive, the kidney action increased, and this in turn cleared the system of that excessive acid condition. In a few weeks the back ceased to ache and pain, as it had done for some time. The arm loosened up and she was able to raise it a few inches higher after each treatment. She was soon able to resume her duties at the switchboard and has been feeling fine ever since.

Neuritis of the Shoulder

I could fill many pages relating the various experiences encountered where the arm and shoulder were lame from some form of neuritis. It may be interesting to relate my experience with one of these.

Case Record

Mr. S., while at his work, fell on a slippery floor, causing a severe injury to his shoulder. He had several X-rays taken which proved there were no broken bones, but the pain grew worse till at the end of three weeks he was unable to sleep without a sedative for the severe pain. He could not raise or move his arm, and he came to me with tears in his eyes as he was suffering so severely and dreaded to see night coming on when it always seemed worse. It was his right shoulder, so I took the right foot and without any further ceremony, reached for the part leading to his lame shoulder. I will admit the tears did not let up, but simply increased as he pleaded for mercy, not that I was harsh or rough, but the tenderness was so extreme even to the slightest touch. As I worked on it, the pain, however, soon let up.

In a case of this kind it is best to work two or three minutes, then rest a little and meanwhile try to convince the patient that this tenderness in his foot is there as a reflex from that experienced in his shoulder, as you want him to be patient with you and your work for fifteen or twenty minutes. Let your conversation be cheerful and constructive to keep his mind off what you are doing as much as possible. In the meantime you are holding his right foot in your left hand using your thumb with pressure to work this reflex as you steady the pressure with your fingers on the top of the foot as in Fig. 20.

Keep working around this joint of the little toe and watch the improvement. By this time he will most likely be able to raise his arm up over his head, as did Mr. S. and it was less than a week when he was able to go back to work.

It is most interesting to work on such cases. Your efforts will be rewarded so quickly and results will be lasting.

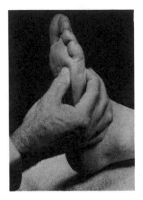

FIGURE 20

**Position for Working the Reflex
to the Shoulder.**

A BROKEN SHOULDER

Case Record

Let me mention here also a case where the shoulder had been broken in an automobile accident, both the clavicle and scapula were broken within an inch of the glenoid cavity, and the humerus was cracked.

The patient, a physician about seventy years of age, was taken to the hospital as he also received a broken leg just below the knee and three fractured ribs, all on the left side. The leg was placed in a cast and the shoulder in a specially formed brace.

He called for me soon after all parts, casts, etc., had been set and adjusted. The part for the shoulder on his left foot was just at the edge of the cast leaving it possible for me to do my part on the reflex for the broken shoulder, which by now was already most tender.

Since he was in such a weakened condition from the seriousness of the accident, it was advisable that I do only a little at a time and that more often. At first I worked it gently a little every day then every second day. It was remarkable to watch the speed of his recovery and the excellent use he soon regained of the arm and shoulder.

It is evident, this method of Reflexology used on that particular reflex hastened the progress and healing of those broken bones by increasing the circulation and relieving the congestion.

TO LOOSEN THE MUSCLES OF THE SHOULDER

We find a large majority of people suffering more or less from a tired feeling across the back of the neck and shoulders. To help relieve this nervous tension, press firmly with the knuckles against the sole of the foot while you work to loosen up the cords and muscles across the top of the foot as shown in Fig. 21.

These will be extremely tight where the patient is nervous and high strung. In such a case do not neglect to work this part thoroughly on each foot, for it will prove a very important factor in bringing about relief from many ailments caused by undue nerve tension.

73

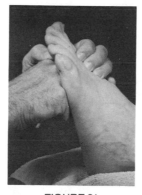

FIGURE 21
**Position for Loosening the Muscles
of the Shoulder and Neck.**

Working this part of the foot is also very essential where there is any tendency to a broken metatarsal arch. If this condition has existed very long, you must be persistent with this reflex work in order to break up and loosen any calcium deposits which may have formed around the joints which have become misplaced.

If any one or more of the 26 bones of the foot should be misplaced, nature fills in that misplaced joint with a calcium deposit which we can help to loosen and dissolve by this form of Reflexology over the top of the foot as shown in Fig. 21, and also the twisting movement as illustrated in Fig. 26.

You will readily see how this will help nature to carry away any such foreign matter which interferes with the normal position of the bones.

A LAME HIP

Keep in mind this reflex in the shoulder where there is a condition in any part of the hip.

Since a reflex can be found in the shoulder for the hip, let us remember that to loosen up any part of the shoulder will have a tendency to relieve tightness and congestion in the hip. It will require a very deep pressure as illustrated in Fig. 21 and Fig. 20.

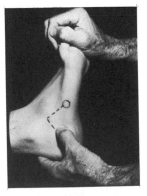

FIGURE 22

**Position for Loosening the Muscles
Relative to Knee, Hip and Lower Back Area.**

Should the pain extend below the hip between that and the knee, deeply reflex that part of the arm between the shoulder and the elbow; any heavy deep massage given around the shoulder and back of the neck will help relieve any tightness or congestion in the corresponding part of the hip.

It is also well to remember the same rule holds good with the shoulder. Many times a pain there can be relieved by deep pressure of the corresponding part in the hip itself. Be sure to work the reflex to the hips as shown in Fig. 22.

Arthritis

Arthritis is a condition from which many are seeking relief. Like every other ailment there must be a cause. If that cause is an infection brought about by food poisoning, let us see why the digestive system is lazy and fails to function normally.

The time occupied for a normal meal to pass through the digestive system (stomach and intestines) is from twelve to eighteen hours, but if these organs are weakened by a congestion in the nerve endings (in the feet), then the stomach fails to function properly.

Food supposed to be acted upon in the stomach, if not properly prepared for its reception into the intestines, ferments and decomposes. The blood, which is dependent upon the material handed to it from the digestive organs, is overloaded with acid or calcium deposits. As this condition increases, the vitality of the body decreases, leaving the patient subject to arthritis, rheumatism, neuritis, etc. Thus if you will seek to find the cause from "The Stories the Feet Can Tell," you will most likely find which organ or organs might be mainly responsible for this condition and, as in everything else, if we can remove the cause we help the effect. Do not look for results in arthritis in a minute, a day or a week. It will take time. They will most likely feel somewhat worse from the first few treatments due to the reaction, but do not become impatient for results. As long as the slightest tenderness remains in the nerve endings in the feet, you are still fighting to break up and scatter crystalline deposits.

Circulation and Constipation

Increased circulation can become a powerful housecleaning agent, and thus stimulate a rectal action in a normal regular rhythm without the use of drugs or the regular old fashioned enema with which in olden times people prided themselves in the number of gallons of water they could use, and the length of time it took to perform this bowel cleansing. At times it has been known that three to eight gallons of water were used and an hour and a half of time consumed.

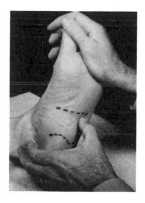

FIGURE 23
Position for Working the Reflex
to the Descending Colon.

We all admit that in cases of acute autointoxication, this method of immediate relief might be necessary, and be used to great advantage. But where the present condition has already existed over a period of time without any serious effects except ordinary discomfort, we can afford to give nature a little time to adjust its elimination, and thus allow the large bowel to serve the useful purpose nature intended it should, by absorbing through its walls some of the water and certain necessary minerals which are returned to the body after entering it from the small intestines. At this point it is in somewhat of a liquid state. As the absorption takes place, the contents of the large lower bowel becomes semi-solid, and to help this mass to pass on with the normal muscular action of the bowels, it must become lubricated with mucus secreted by the intestinal glands, and finally it reaches the rectum almost solid.

Here we need proper contraction of the muscles in the walls of the large bowel to call the attention of the person to the fact that he is ready for a movement.

You can readily see that any change in this program brought about by the habitual use of a purgative or an irritating enema, will change the natural routine nature mapped out. Don't try to improve on God's natural laws of nature. It is only as we abuse these precious laws that we suffer from the many ills mankind has fallen heir to.

Relaxing Effect

SOME CASES OF CONSTIPATION

It is very evident from the results we obtain, that this method of Reflexology treatment has a definite relaxing influence on the part being treated through the reflex. You will come to the same conclusion with me, after having a few experiences similar to what I have had in some cases of constipation.

CONSTIPATION AND CONTRACTION

Now since the cause of this prevailing ailment is often due to a contraction or tension of some form of the lower bowel, we find that we should thoroughly work the area on the inner side of each ankle, beginning from the heel and working up about six or eight inches, will often produce an immediate bowel movement. For location see Fig. 24.

The position of the hands in giving this treatment is the same as described for disorders of the rectum.

We can also emphasize this effect by loosening up the tendon of Achilles, the cord leading up the back of the leg from the heel. You may do this while the foot is still in the firm grasp of your hand. It will feel much like a firm rubber cord. While you are using the tips of your fingers for the other work we have described, do not fail at the same time to press this cord back and forth in any way that might tend to stretch it and relieve any form of tightness, hold the ankle firmly while twisting the foot as shown in Fig. 26.

JUST WHEN TO EXPECT IMMEDIATE RESULTS

Do not misunderstand me and say I claim that every form of constipation can be relieved by this method. I qualified it, in the beginning of this chapter, when I said some cases of constipation are due to nerve tension affecting and tightening the sphincter muscles of the rectum causing undue contraction of the sigmoid flexure.

It is with cases of this origin we so often obtain immediate results. It is nothing unusual to have someone come into my office, and rave about how much good I have done for them and their particular case of constipation. Perhaps since the first Reflexology treatment they have been able to discard the use of their daily cathartic, while the neighbor next door may fail to respond till the whole intestinal tract, liver, and gall bladder have been brought into proper action.

LENGTH OF TIME

The length of time for results in a case of this kind will depend entirely on just how long they have been in getting out of tune, or whether they may have had one or more operations to impede the progress of this repair work. Perhaps, too, they have had their appendix removed, robbing the intestines of that little oil supply so important to the normal action of the bowels.

We who have been fortunate enough to escape any such operation, robbing us of any organ of our body, however small or insignificant it may seem, have just that much more for which to be thankful. We will also be in a condition to respond more readily to REFLEXOLOGY treatments.

Rectal Disorders

It is astonishing the results that can be obtained from this treatment for various disorders of the rectum. We will first give you the location of this reflex. Stop and think and in your mind's eye decide in which zone the rectum is located. Being in the center of the body, places it in the first zone. Therefore, we will find this reflex on the inner side of each ankle about half an inch from the cord leading up the back of the leg, shown in Fig. 24.

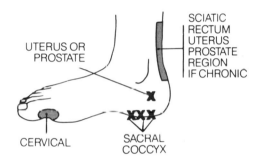

FIGURE 24

The tenderness here may extend three to five inches up from the heel, according to the amount and location of the trouble in the rectum, which varies in length from six to eight inches.

This will be found extremely tender, wherever there is an inflamed or abnormal condition of the rectum.

Prostate Gland

We find the location of this important gland, which resembles that of a horsechestnut in form and size, is in the first zone, since it surrounds the neck of the bladder and commencement of the urethra, lying in the pelvic cavity behind and below the symphisis pubis upon the rectum. An enlargement of this gland will cause considerable pain and inconvenience and often results in a great deal of difficulty in voiding the urine. It affects the nervous system and is oftentimes responsible for the patient being aroused a number of times during the night to urinate.

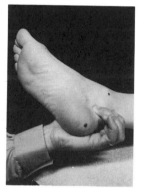

FIGURE 25

**Position for Working the Reflex
to the Prostate Gland on Both Feet.**

Wherever this condition exists you will be sure to find this reflex to the rectum very tender, perhaps extending down to the lower part of the inside of the heel toward that of the bladder. Lying so closely together it is impossible to separate the reflex, but you will find a tenderness here at this point to tell of the congestion to that particular part or gland which is causing the inflammation or irritation.

AN ENLARGED PROSTATE GLAND

First find the location as per Fig. 24 and Fig. 25.

After locating the tenderness, grasp the foot according to directions given for treating disorders of the rectum.

Continue the pressure and creeping motion with the thumb or finger tips, using whichever seems the best way to work out and dissolve the crystal-like substance that has accumulated in that particular nerve ending, caused by the inflammation and enlargement of the gland.

Remember you are endeavoring to restore the normal circulation without any direct contact which would tend to set up an increased irritation. There has been a cause for this gland to grow into a diseased state, and that cause was no doubt a congestion brought about by the crystals in these nerve endings.

Now let us consider how we can cause this gland to grow out of this diseased condition. Certainly there is no better or more effective way to do this, than to supply the parts again with the amount of free and normal circulation nature intended they should have.

Case Record

To prove this statement I shall relate a case that came to my attention a little while ago. Mr. V., a man about 50 years of age, had been having treatments for an enlarged prostate gland, with little or no results. I proceeded at once with this Reflex method in the manner as shown in Fig. 25. I found as I always do in such cases, a great deal of tenderness in the reflex to the prostate gland. But after the tenderness had been completely worked out we found the trouble had entirely disappeared, and instead of being disturbed from four to six times each night to urinate, he was able to rest undisturbed for eight or ten hours.

Now at this time there happened a most interesting coincidence. For some time Mr. V. had been conscious that a small growth had formed just inside at the end of the rectum which he was very anxious to have removed. Since he was now feeling in the pink of condition he thought it a most opportune time to have this slight operation performed.

The Reflexology treatments I had given him had completely cleared up all the tenderness of that part, and relieved all undue congestion from the prostate gland. His nervousness had improved too. The night before the operation we tested it out thoroughly to assure ourselves that not the slightest tenderness anywhere remained.

Then I arranged to see Mr. V. again as soon as possible following the operation. At this time I knew we would find an exaggerated amount of tenderness in the lower part of the ankle as the result of the operation, which as I explained to Mr. V. would be a splendid test as to the accuracy of my statements, and the location of the reflexes.

When I arrived he had only been home a few hours from the doctor's office. He was in considerable pain with the rectum aching and throbbing and feeling very uncomfortable. I immediately found the reflex with the tip of my third finger, and to him it felt, under the slightest pressure, as if I were piercing it with a piece of broken glass; the same place and tenderness showing up on each ankle.

It is evident the removal of this growth directly on the rectum, which is the center of the body, had affected the first zone on each side.

I proceeded with gentle pressure on first one ankle, then the other, alternating about every two minutes for about a quarter of an hour. The throbbing soon disappeared and it was amazing the amount of relief this gave him and so soon, even following an operation. He was able at once to turn over in bed without pain, and was up and around as usual in a short time.

Hemorrhoids

We will now consider a case of hemorrhoids (commonly called piles). This is a condition of varicose veins (congestion) in the rectum, causing very great tenderness and inconvenience, and sometimes bleeding. It is on account of this tenderness in the region of the rectum that we find the reflex to the rectum so sensitive, indicating a congestion preventing the circulation.

ONE POSITION FOR TREATING HEMORRHOIDS

As you sit facing the patient, first place the left heel in your left hand, grasp the leg with your right hand just above the ankle from the under side. With the tips of your fingers pointing upward, hold the foot steady with your left hand. You must use the right hand to work firmly with a rotary motion, till you locate the tenderest spot, and there continue with your pressure, and working in the same way and in the same place as that outlined for disorders of the rectum. Reverse the procedure on the right heel.

NOT TOO MUCH PRESSURE

You must use caution not to be too severe, the nerves being close to the surface at this point. It will require time and patience more than severity.

Let me say again, you must watch the expression of your patient carefully to determine just where and when you are reaching the point that will produce the desired effect (tenderness). So often the beginner will keep watching his hands. Learn to let the hands automatically hunt and find the sore places without trying to look at them. It is far more important to watch the expression attentively, which helps you to determine how much pressure can be used without causing too much pain.

You are not trying to do the work all in a minute. It will require time. As you see the distress signal on the face of the patient, caused by what you are doing, you can let up quickly and proceed more gently and can also locate your reflex more correctly. This reflex may cover only an area as large as a pea, and sometimes even less.

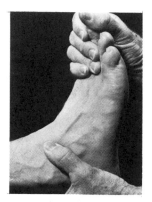

FIGURE 26

Method of Twisting Foot for Relief of Congestion in General.

In a condition of hemorrhoids you will find a tightness of the heavy cord leading up the back of the leg, which may be loosened up considerably by twisting the foot around in a circulatory motion three or four times to the right, then alternating three or four times to the left, pulling the heel and stretching the cord by pressing the foot forward and pulling it backward. This can be done best while the foot is still in this position with the heel resting on your hand.

I want to say here that before giving this twist you must change the grasp of your right hand to that of the top of the foot, as shown in Fig. 26. The more pressure placed by the heel of your right hand against the sole of the foot, at the location of the metatarsal arch, while twisting the foot, the greater the tendency to loosen up the bones and correct any slight misplacement that might exist in that particular arch. This work done faithfully twice a week allowing about one half hour for each treatment till all tenderness had disappeared will practically remove all discomfort and annoyance caused by any case of hemorrhoids.

CASE RECORD

It may be interesting here to relate an experience I had in Miami, Florida, a few years ago, I was explaining this method of treating, and how we could locate the reflex to the rectum etc. to a small group of friends, when a young lady stepped forward whom I had never met before and offered herself as a subject for me to use in demonstrating this method of REFLEXOLOGY

Her outward appearance was that of perfect health, so I began the examination in the usual way, wondering if I would be able to find any tender reflex to indicate any weakness in one so apparently healthy.

Beginning at the big toe I proceeded with the usual pressure on each of the principal reflexes of the foot, without the slightest response to indicate any tenderness or bodily ailment. But as I grasped the ankle and began to press on the point which would indicate some rectal disorder, or most likely hemorrhoids, she almost jumped out of the chair and exclaimed, "Oh, that hurts!"

Knowing I had located some ailment or weakness I went on to ask the young lady if she might have had any trouble in that line recently. Before answering me, she smiled as if to ask, "How did I know?"—then went onto tell that only a few weeks before, she had undergone the third operation for hemorrhoids and had not yet entirely recovered.

She was most thoroughly convinced with the truthfulness of my remarks. What interested us all still further was the story she went on to tell. As she was "coming to" from the effects of the anesthetic given for her last operation, before gaining consciousness, she had to be strapped to the bed to prevent her from constantly rising up and grabbing her heels and crying, "Oh, how my heels hurt."

KNOWLEDGE OF "REFLEXOLOGY"

With the knowledge we have now of the zones and reflexes of the body we can readily understand why nature was calling out in despair at the damage done to some part of that elementary nerve canal zone. While the mind was still in that state of semi-consciousness, the sub-conscious mind was working and calling for pressure to that reflex as a form of relief.

Had the nurses in that hospital understood REFLEX-OLOGY and instead of strapping her down in bed, had administered Reflex Therapy to that region of her heel, it would have given this poor girl a great deal of relief, and would have aided the process of recovery by increasing the circulation to the wounded area.

Suffice to say, from this demonstration the young lady was a firm believer in REFLEXOLOGY. She placed herself in my care for a while and she was soon feeling fit and fine as ever.

PROLAPSED RECTUM

Case Record

As further evidence of what can really be accomplished by work of this kind I will relate a case I had the pleasure of caring for in my own family.

A lady over 70 years of age, since the birth of her daughter some 30 years ago, had been troubled terribly with a prolapsed rectum. Each year as she grew older, it became worse and protruded more and more. A greater portion of the time it would be swollen badly and very much inflamed.

A number of physicians had suggested an operation, as a means of the only possible relief, it being very likely to produce even a more serious form of trouble by destroying the muscular action of the rectum for all future time.

Knowing a little experimentation on my part with our Reflex work would do no harm, I set out to see what I could do. The results and the benefit that she received from a few of these treatments were almost unbelievable. The inflammation and swelling subsided entirely, and it has caused her little or no trouble since. I simply used the method I have outlined for disorders of the rectum and hemorrhoids.

Let me say here that in this case the tenderness was extremely manifest and many times she would plead for mercy during the treatment, when in reality the pressure was in no way severe. But as the tenderness gradually worked out the condition improved.

Inflammation of the Bladder

CYSTITIS

Inflammation of the bladder causing a frequent desire to urinate, is a condition very easy to handle with this form of treatment. The reflex is found on each foot, in practically the same location as outlined for the lower part of rectum only a little more toward and under the ankle bone as in Fig. 27. The bladder and rectum being in so nearly the same (first) zone. This works out quickly, perhaps the second or third treatment will show a marked improvement, together with your work on the kidneys which will help to lessen the formation of uric acid which no doubt originally was caused by cystitis.

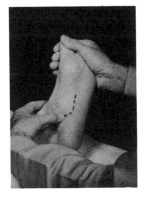

FIGURE 27

**Method for Working the Reflex
to the Bladder and Ureter.**

Tension of
Female Organs

UTERUS

It is with this same mode of treatment that you will be able to help many a trouble caused by a tension or a tightening of the muscles of the uterus and vagina. This condition is responsible for a great deal of nervousness and the breaking up of many a happy home.

When a case of this kind is brought to your attention, think a little of what might be the cause and effect, and set out to remedy it. Perhaps you will be able to steer more than one unhappy individual from the rocks of disaster.

OVARIES

Now picture in your mind the location of the ovaries. They are located somewhat away from the center and each one off to the side a little. Thus we will find the reflex to the right ovary on the outside of the right heel, and the left ovary reflected on the outside of the left heel. Fig. 28.

Where the thyroid gland is affected in any way, you will most likely find this point tender too, as the thyroid gland is considered sort of a third ovary, and connected very closely in their relationship to the functioning of the monthly period.

I could relate some wonderful results I have had in this line, where the irregularity was caused by an abnormal functioning of the thyroid gland.

Case Record

One case I remember in particular, a young lady 35 years old had never menstruated regularly since maturity.

Instead of the normal period every twenty-eight days she was always exactly forty days between her periods. She had, since childhood, been subject to severe attacks of hives, considered most likely the result of a nervous disturbance of some form. Finally she began to lose interest in her home, did not care to live, lost weight rapidly, went down from 130 pounds to about 90 pounds.

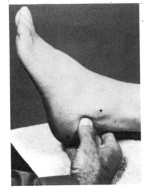

FIGURE 28

**Position for Working the
Left Ovary.**

She was taken to the hospital for observation. Tests showed a case of exophthalmic goitre. She was ordered to return home and build up for the operation they advised. She came to me at this time.

I found a great deal of nerve tension and congestion present in the location just outlined for ailments of this kind. She was persuaded to postpone the operation and give me a chance to see what could be done with this reflex work.

Improvement was noticeable almost immediately from the beginning of the treatments. Her nerves improved, she grew more calm every day, rested better, and as I recall, it was only two or three weeks till she began to gain weight regularly, about one pound a week, till she was again back to normal, feeling like herself and in splendid condition. She was now for the first time in her life normal and regular in her monthly periods, proving what I am trying to bring out, that a sick thyroid will affect the functioning of the ovaries.

You will often be asked if with this method of Reflexology you can do anything to relieve cramps during the menstruation period. In a case where the cause is congestion you will get surprising results. We all know there may be a variety of causes for a condition of this kind.

While we do not claim this method to be any form of magic, or a cure-all for every ailment let us not fail to give it credit for what we know it can do for such a large variety of cases. Let us consider a case of hemorrhage. I would say, by all means, do not give this treatment during that period, unless guided and directed by a competent physician familiar with the case and familiar with the results obtainable from this Reflex Therapy treatment.

RESULTS WILL FOLLOW

By your persistent endeavor you will be sure to obtain results, and these various ailments will finally disappear. Not overnight, nor in a day, nor a week, as you must remind the patient, this is not a faith cure performed by wielding some magic wand over the head, but a scientific method worked out on scientific principles.

Our body is constructed to endure a lot of abuse. We have been breaking the laws of nature over a period of months and years, and it will take time to rebuild and replace these sick broken down cells.

93

We are inclined to give the working of our automobile more thought and consideration than we do our precious body. We take it to a garage every now and then for a checkup, to see that every bolt and nut is tight, and that every part is properly lubricated, even the slightest rattle or squeak receives our immediate attention. But when a pain attacks us here and there, as a warning of some impending danger, we try to brush it aside and say, "Oh, it will wear off." Sometimes it will, all well and good, again it may wear us out during the procedure.

How many can we recall who have gone to an earlier grave than necessary because they neglected the danger signal in time to avert the fatal accident, which might have at least been postponed for several years, with a little added attention given to the congested areas of their body?

We must remember circulation is life; stagnation is death; a heavy blow causes congestion, and tenderness is the result. Just so with any part of the body starved by congestion in any part of the zone leading to that particular muscle or organ of the body.

Reflexes Other
Than Found In the Feet

From the teachings set forth and brought out on ZONE THERAPY by Doctor Fitzgerald, we have learned, too, of other reflexes than those found in the feet, which have a lot to do with one being successful in this great cause; a knowledge of which when combined with this work on the feet, can bring relief to many a swollen aching joint.

We who are trained in the science of massage, know very well how often it is inadvisable to massage directly over an aching swollen part, for if a condition of neuritis (inflammation of the nerves) should exist, we might aggravate the trouble and increase the pain. But if we are familiar with the location of the reflex to that particular part in another place on the body, we can work this most thoroughly and have a definite effect on the afflicted area.

Suppose someone comes to you with neuritis in the right knee. You will take the right elbow, and in the exact location on the elbow as that of the trouble in the knee, you will find a tenderness. Work this deeply with the thumb and tips of your fingers, reaching in to loosen up the ligaments, tendons, etc. After keeping this up for perhaps ten minutes, then ask if any improvement is noticed in the condition of the knee; invariably it will be noticeable immediately.

95

Now if the trouble is in the elbow, we work the knee on the same side, which will have a reflex action on the elbow.

We find the wrist can be successfully worked for troubles in the ankle; the right wrist for the right ankle, the left wrist for the left ankle. As in the knee and the elbow so the tenderness will be found in the wrist, in exact proportion corresponding to the location of the tenderness in the ankle.

A STIFF OR LAME SHOULDER

A lame shoulder which will have a particular point of tenderness, can be reached by locating this same point in the hip and working directly on that part of the hip.

A stiffness caused by adhesions following a broken hip, can be greatly improved by deep heavy massage of every muscle in the shoulder on that particular side.

The same method will hold good with a case where the shoulder has been broken, remaining stiff and lame from the effects of a cast or adhesions.

It may be impossible to move the arm, yet the leg and hip on that side can be moved without causing any discomfort. So the work you would like to be doing on the arm and shoulder itself, to loosen it up, but find yourself unable to on account of the stiffness, you can do to the leg and hip on that side and watch the results. You will not be causing any pain yet producing an effect impossible to get by any direct contact with the part itself.

A few experiences in this line will increase your faith and confidence in what can be done with reflex work. Some improvements will be observed and felt almost immediately, which encourages both the patient and the operator, and increases faith all around in the effectiveness of what is being done. You may not have to wait for results when you use this method for trouble in the joints, etc.

Mind and Digestion

The state of mind affects digestion more than almost any other bodily ailment.

Constipation is often a state of mind. Dr. Boris Kaplan has published recent studies indicating that financial troubles may cause stomach disorders, which become ulcers. The worries affect the digestion, and the digestive troubles increase the worry. Thus, a case refusing to respond to the usual form of this foot treatment, may be traced to some emotional disturbance in the patient's life.

I will relate a case here that was brought to my attention. Mrs. H., about 45 years of age, came to me for treatments. Her husband was a very successful business man and had always been a good provider. She had a comfortable home, a cottage at the lake in the summer, and four nice children, youngest still in high school. But in spite of it all, she developed a complex which led her to believe she was sick. She visited several physicians, who with X-rays and various tests, could discover nothing wrong with her condition, for which they were heartily condemned. Her husband, frantic to find help, brought her to me, as a last resort, and as I began to explain my method of finding a tenderness in the reflex of the foot, leading to the affected part, she began to tell me she knew she had colitis, and ulcers of the stomach. She couldn't eat, she couldn't sleep, and she knew she was going to lose her mind if something could not be done for her.

From the sound of her story I expected to find a number of tender places. As I now proceeded with the usual procedure, to my surprise I too found nothing to indicate any calcium or crystal deposits, which would instead prove a very healthy condition, verifying the physician's diagnosis. Her husband, believing my method to be his last resort, insisted I try to convince her that it would be of some help. On each visit, she would assure me she was going to lose her mind, as she was so very sick. I used all the power of suggestion that was possible to bring to bear, but to no avail. Nothing I could do helped her because there was no real trouble to correct, except the mental complex which was so deeply rooted in her mind, that she brought upon herself the very mental condition she feared. And in a short time it was necessary to confine her to the State Hospital, where she has been for the last two years.

How pitiful to see anyone bring about such a condition simply from a distorted mental attitude, when no real physical ailment existed. Without a doubt, Mrs. H. attracted to herself that which she actually feared. As we continue our study along this line, we find that most bodily ailments affect us in proportion as we give them attention.

There is not an organ in the body that is not affected by the mind. Every thought we think either has a constructive or a destructive reaction on the chemical content of our blood stream. We cannot let thoughts of fear, worry, anxiety or grief overcome us without increasing the acidity of our bloodstream. Worry is a magnified form of fear, an idea by which we torment ourselves, a fixation of attention.

How often our health is controlled by fixed ideas. Most of our nervous derangements are brought on by uncontrolled emotions. A suggestion can sometimes prove a power to determine a destiny. Are we going to let thoughts of fear kill the cells of our body? How many times have we seen the seriousness of an epidemic increased by the fear thoughts that invaded the minds of people? The twenty-seven trillion cells of the body all have their thinking machine, and they all respond to the law of suggestion. It is the law of creation, and we cannot tamper with it.

CIRCULATION FOLLOWS ATTENTION

A doctor who breezes into a sick room with a cheerful disposition, can do a world of good for his patient, and can start the creative powers to work, or he can have the opposite effect. for those who are down and sick are always susceptible to suggestion.

It is an acknowledged fact that the body is affected by the mind. Every flitting change of the mind causes a chemical change in the body. Circulation follows attention. We are told that the center of every cell in the body is composed of the same grey matter as the brain. Every time we think a thought, we use up energy. Then why continue to poison our system and waste our energies by harboring destructive thoughts of fear, worry, envy, jealousy and their kindred folks? We cannot change a natural law. It takes certain laws and principles to make us free from disease. And the more we learn of the truth about the laws of nature, that rule and govern our health—which too are also God's laws—the quicker our system becomes freed from these destructive agencies, and we no longer continue in such a way as to tear down our body cells.

Mind and Demand

Our mind can change a demand. Our ideals can be changed by a new thought. Some authorities go so far as to claim that cancer can be caused by a long continuous nerve retention. That gall bladder trouble can be brought on by anxiety; that secretive nervous irritation can cause fibroid tumor; and constipation can be brought on by obstinacy, and some forms of rheumatism to be a state of unconscious unwillingness to face the problems of life. Whether this will all be true or not, we mention it for your consideration. No doubt the predominant mental impression is what governs the mind and the functioning of every part of our being even to the tiniest cell.

CRYSTALLINE DEPOSITS

This in turn has to do with governing the acid content in our bloodstream, and the amount of crystals that may be liable to form in the nerve ending of any organ of the body that might be unable to do its part in keeping up with the normal muscular action necessary to keep the circulation normally perfect.

If the gas line in our automobile becomes choked up in any way, the carburetor ceases to function properly, and the power dies down. Then we must go to a garage, and employ the aid of someone trained in locating the obstruction to eliminate it.

ACID DEPOSITS

This corresponds exactly with the work we are aiming to do to these acid deposits in the nerve endings of the feet. We must clear the gas line (arteries and veins) of any foreign obstruction, before the carburetor (heart) can work proficiently and furnish the body sufficient power and pep to perform its round of duty as nature intended it should. Since we cannot exchange this old body for a new model every year, it is all the more necessary that we give special attention to the one and only one we can ever own.

OUR BODY A MACHINE

This machine, our body, is one thing left to our care, and if we abuse it, the sooner it will wear out.

If we allow calcium deposits to increase in our arteries after the age of forty, we are soon having high blood pressure, overburdening the heart in its effort to keep the blood in circulation even to the tiniest nerve extremities of the hands and feet.

What Is Pain?

Pain is not a disease, but it is true indication of a disturbance, a congestion in some part or parts. Pain is not an evil but a blessing, calling out for help; a cry of nature. Then why try to deaden the warning call by the use of aspirin or some sedative which will only tend to paralyze the nerve centers and lessen our chances to locate the trouble. Dr. Chapman has very well said, "Pain is the cry of a hungry nerve for better blood supply." And we say, yes, for better weapons to fight for perfect circulation, despite the various obstructions along the nerve channel and nerve endings where pain can be traced and found with the slightest pressure. We may take a person in perfect health with a perfect circulatory system and find no pain whatever in spite of all the pressure you can possibly bring to bear on any part of the foot. You will meet a few really healthy individuals, but they are few and far between, for it seems that the majority of mankind have some form of an ailment.

ONE HEALTHY YOUNG MAN

I was invited to dinner one evening by a patient of mine whose son from Buffalo was to be present. His mother, Mrs. C., tried to impress me with the idea that she was greatly worried over his condition, the nature of which she would not reveal, but left me to find where the trouble might be. As I proceeded in the usual way, trying various reflexes, I found not the slightest tenderness anywhere. I did not wish to disappoint Mr. C. or myself by being unable to locate the trouble, so after a most thorough tryout I had to give up, and in a way holding my breath said, "You really must be in perfect health." At this remark I was soon relieved to see the whole family smile and assure me that this occasion had been planned as a test case to see if this method was correct. Only a week before Mr. C. has passed an examination for a twenty thousand dollar Life Insurance policy with the company's compliments on his unusually wonderful health.

It is interesting to encounter experiences similar to this. So often people think their feet are perfectly well, and will say to you, "Oh, my feet are the best part of me." The real fact is, their bodily ailments have not yet been realized, only in the form of an occasional headache, or perhaps some indigestion now and then, which nature has sent out in the form of a danger signal.

VARIOUS METHODS

Remember there are many successful methods of helping various ailments. The physician can often give a pill or write a prescription containing some herb extraction equalizing the acidity, or alkalinity of the blood stream. This increases the vitality of the body sufficiently to rid these nerve extremities of any obstruction caused by an acid formation, without the method outlined in this book. But it is an indisputable fact that we can help nature to perform her important duties more efficiently and obtain quicker and more lasting results along any line of practice by the addition of this simple method of Reflexology herein outlined, which can be administered successfully by any nurse or attendant.

Importance of Proper Circulation

Every practitioner will admit the importance of proper circulation in order to have a body free from congestion and the hundred and one ailments caused from this condition. No one can deny the well known fact that circulation is life; stagnation is death. As long as any part of the one hundred percent normal circulation is being cut off from any one or more parts of the body, be it only that of a tiny gland, we begin to feel the effect in one way or another; with a pain here or an ache there. Nature tries to cry out and tell us these various defects in time to remedy them, but we pay no attention and try to silence the alarm with some deadening pill. But as a chain is no stronger than its weakest link, so our body is no stronger than its weakest point.

Now remember nature will do her part if we give her half a chance. So if we can learn some simple way to stimulate the normal circulation by relieving the congestion in the various nerve endings in the feet, is it not worth some careful consideration? I do not ask you to believe something that has not been already proven beyond any doubt; I only ask you to try it out for yourself, and watch for results.

A CONCLUDING THOUGHT

In concluding this work on "Stories The Feet Can Tell," let me remind you again that Reflexology in any form is only a means of exercise, a means of equalizing the circulation.

We all know circulation is life. Stagnation is death. Everything around us that is alive is in motion.

Everything in the universe is governed by the law of motion, which is one of God's great infallible laws of nature. It is from the earth, sun, and water which are constantly in motion that we receive our creative forces which are followed by growth, maturity and decay. Nothing stands still. Our vitality is either increasing or decreasing according to the quality and circulation of our bloodstream.

Study for a moment the life of a sturdy oak, which from a tiny acorn grows. Stop and observe how it lifts its leafy arms toward Heaven to receive from the passing breezes the exercise necessary to strengthen its root supply, increasing the capacity to gather moisture and nourishment necessary to furnish and keep the sap flowing freely through every part. If we cut off the roots sufficiently to rob it of its life-giving sap, how long will the tree be green and full of life?

In the face of this shall we forget the necessity of keeping our whole body in motion; every part in perfect rhythm.

It is my sincere wish that this new technique of FOOT REFLEXOLOGY will stand side by side with other great therapy works in the onward march of science and progress.

EUNICE D. INGHAM

STORIES
THE FEET
HAVE TOLD

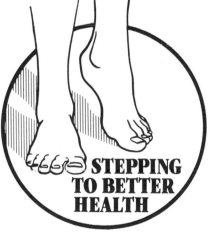

STEPPING
TO BETTER
HEALTH

REFLEXOLOGY

Zone Therapy
and
Gland Reflexes

*"Look! 'tis the feet of a herald,
hastening over the hills, with glad,
good news, with tidings of relief."*
                    ISAIAH 52-7 (Moffatt)

Preface

In the pages to follow, I shall endeavor to present a detailed account of the INGHAM COMPRESSION METHOD OF REFLEXOLOGY.

It is a method acknowledged at the present time throughout the country by men of authority as a scientific approach to a particular form of specialized tissue manipulation influencing nerve impulses in the feet, creating added relaxation invaluable to the profession.

Why not seek to be among those who have won distinctive recognition and well-deserved fame in the field of manipulative therapy? Let us light our candle from theirs and may the benediction of the masters bless our efforts.

Since great oaks from little acorns grow, it is my hope that the seed planted by the thoughts herein set forth will take root in fertile soil and grow for the benefit and relief of suffering humanity.

EUNICE INGHAM STOPFEL

i

What Is this Reflex Method?

There are ten zone areas in the body that furnish us a general principle for finding certain reflexes in the feet.

Will a new profession relative to these reflexes in the human foot originate?

The most talked about yet least understood topic in the profession today.

DR. OSLER'S STATEMENT
"When the nerves of the eyes and the feet are properly understood there will be less need for surgical intervention."

Fools Deride Where Philosophers Investigate

Ingham Compression Method of Reflexology

ITS APPLICATION TO THE GLANDS AND KINDRED AILMENTS

In answer to numerous requests, I shall endeavor to set forth in print a more detailed account of how to apply my particular reflex method for greater and better results in relieving ailments caused by some abnormal glandular activity.

It is almost impossible to realize the importance of each tiny gland, as our knowledge and the facts of the enormous power of hormone secretion are so limited.

ELECTRICAL SYSTEM

The nerves of our body may be likened to an electrical system. It will be our ability to make the normal contact with the electricity in the ground, through our feet and from the elements or atmosphere surrounding us, that will determine the degree of power we are able to manifest in the proper functioning of these glands.

Trying to get a normal contact where there is congestion in these nerve terminals in the feet is like trying to put a plug into a defective fixture.

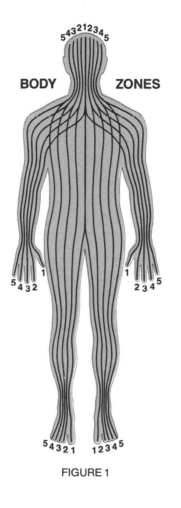

BODY ZONES

FIGURE 1

A study of this diagram will graphically place in the mind the zones of the body.

As there are ten fingers and ten toes we may conceive ten zones of the limbs and all parts of the body.

WHAT IS ZONE THERAPY

It is a principle of dividing the body into ten zones, aiding us in our ability to locate the reflexes in the feet relative to every part of the body.

Zone Therapy

Let us analyze the term ZONE THERAPY in connection with our reflex work, which has been misunderstood and is meaningless without a better knowledge of what it stands for in the way of a directional guide in locating the specific reflexes we are trying to find and contact.

The medical dictionary in defining the word zone gives as an explanatory example: "Abdominal zone, the three zones into which the surface of the abdomen is divided by the subcostal and intertubercular lines."

Let us keep this same principle in mind as to what we mean by the term ZONE THERAPY as our guiding principle for locating certain reflex areas.

One who is not familiar with its proper meaning will immediately assume we are advancing something entirely different from the simple reflex method outlined in my books *"STORIES THE FEET CAN TELL"* and *"STORIES THE FEET HAVE TOLD."*

International Institute of Reflexology®
presents
Advanced Ingham Method™ Seminars

- **Theory, Demonstration and Instruction** based on over 55 years of research and teaching are combined in a complete Seminar to give you the best possible instruction in the art of Foot Reflexology.

- These seminars are taught with a combination of multi-media training aids ranging from film graphics to individualized physical application, in order to give you a firm preliminary foundation in Reflexology techniques.

- Most important are our authorized, qualified instructors. We have found there are many individuals attempting to pass themselves off as I.I.R. qualified instructors teaching the Original Ingham Method™. They may have attended our seminars, but that does not compare to the training of our instructors. If you have any questions regarding an instructor, please call the I.I.R. at (813) 343-4811.

See reverse side of this card for location nearest you.

The International Institute of Reflexology®
and
Ingham Publishing
presents
The Original Ingham Method™ of Foot Reflexology

Please send me FREE INFORMATION regarding...

☐ **Books and charts available**   ☐ **Seminars in my area**

NAME _____

ADDRESS _____

CITY _____ STATE _____

POST. CODE _____ COUNTRY _____
Rev. 2/96

Be Sure To Read...

The original works of Eunice D. Ingham
**"STORIES THE FEET CAN TELL THRU REFLEXOLOGY /
STORIES THE FEET HAVE TOLD THRU REFLEXOLOGY"**

with revisions by
The World's Leading Authority on Foot Reflexology...
Dwight C. Byers
Nephew of Eunice Ingham

Don't Delay – Send For More Information Today!

Learn More Through The Seminars
**Presented Annually in
The United States, Canada, Great Britain,
Ireland, Europe, Israel, Australia,
New Zealand, South Africa and Asia**

● For further information mail the card below — TODAY! Your name and
address will be directed to the Seminar Director for your area.
Or Call 813-343-4811
P.O. BOX 12642, ST. PETERSBURG, FLORIDA 33733 U.S.A.

PLACE
STAMP
HERE

**International Institute of Reflexology
P.O. Box 12642
St. Petersburg, Florida 33733-2642
U.S.A.**

What Is Zone Therapy
Via the Reflexes?

I hope the pages to follow will answer satisfactorily the question WHAT IS ZONE THERAPY? and its relation to the reflex method herein set forth, as we try to prove beyond all doubt that there does exist a reflex area in the feet relative to every organ and part of the body.

Now we must aim to increase our ability to determine accurately the location of these various reflexes. This will be dependent upon our knowledge of the governing principle of how the body can be visualized into ten particular zones, five on the right side and five on the left side of the body, both anterior and posterior.

To this valuable principle we owe the credit for methods recommended, not only in this book, but the one preceding it, entitled *"STORIES THE FEET CAN TELL."* And to this we owe all the success we have had with this method, a way of working with nature so nature will work with us.

Gland Reflexes in the Feet

We are familiar with what stories the spine can tell us as we learn from day to day of the wonderful work being accomplished by those trained in that particular profession.

It has remained for us who are skilled in the art of this method to bring to your attention the wonderful results of WHAT STORIES THE FEET CAN BE MADE TO TELL by applying this particular form of reflexology to the various reflexes in the feet, according to the principles of ZONE THERAPY as discovered and outlined by the late William H. Fitzgerald, M.D.

His discovery of these ten zone areas of the body was brought to the attention of the medical profession in 1913. He pointed out the fact that pressure and stroking of certain zones have a definite effect in bringing about normal functioning in all parts of any specific zone, no matter how remote this area may be from the part upon which the pressure is exerted.

He divided the body into ten longitudinal zones, five on each side of the median line of the body. His theory is that these zones have their origin in the thumb and the first, second, third and fourth fingers, running up the hand and arm, over the face and head, down the front and back of the body, ending in the foot and toes which correspond with the hand and fingers.

His explanation of results obtained is that the human body is an electro-mechanism. Our knowledge of his discovery regarding these ten zone areas gives us a key for accuracy in locating the various reflexes in the feet, which we have discovered affect the terminal areas.

CONTRACTION AND RELAXATION

If every tiny cell is contracting and relaxing as nature

intended it should, we have perfect health and perfect feet. However, let any congestion take place in any part to interfere with that 100 per cent contraction and relaxation, and what do we find?

Suppose by wrong living some gland has become sluggish, the normal contraction and relaxation are lessened. The nerve reflex area to that particular organ, which we find located in the foot, will be tender, telling us in no uncertain terms the story that trouble is there.

At the present time the assumption is that this tenderness is caused by the irritation of crystalline deposits in the area of the nerve reflex of any affected part and that this tenderness is brought about by improper circulation of the fluids to and from the feet relative to the capillary system.

NATURE WILL DO HER PART

Nature will do her part if we can help her by maintaining a normal circulatory system. We are all aware of the fact that circulation is life, stagnation is death. So if we learn some simple way to stimulate the circulation by relieving the congestion in the various areas of the nerve reflexes in the feet, is it not worth our careful investigation?

Let the cause of these tender reflexes be what it may, we are here to discuss what happens when this method of Reflexology is used and the tenderness worked out.

If to every part and organ of the body we find a reflex in the feet, then the extent to which any organ is functioning properly can be determined, by the tenderness this technique reveals on that particular reflex.

If upon pressure of certain areas of the feet the person feels pain, we know the corresponding organ is affected.

If the kidneys are affected, you will find that the kidney reflex will be tender in direct proportion to the amount, and possibly the size, of the crystals and the length of time they have been accumulating.

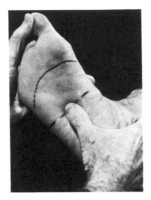

FIGURE 2
Position for Working the Reflex to the Kidneys.

As we use this reflex method on the affected areas, tenderness gradually disappears. The affected organs will again be able to function normally and the patient's symptoms will disappear.

Dizziness

We are often asked what effect this Reflexology Theory may have in relieving dizziness. First try to determine the cause; see what story the liver and gall bladder reflexes may have to tell. Do not forget what goes on in the area of our ears. The inner side of the ear drum contains tubes (semi-circular canals) filled with fluid, and any interference with the normal function of this fluid may lead to the disorder of the body balance causing dizziness, nausea, seasickness, etc., so do not forget the reflex area to the ears when trying to relieve a condition of vertigo, dizziness and/or loss of balance.

Complexity of Reflexes

Remember pain is nature's way of telling us that trouble is at hand.

It is hard to realize fully the complexity of these reflexes. However, no one will deny that any foreign deposits would tend to disorganize the nerve impulses, not only in the feet, but in any part of the body.

If a thought set in motion never ceases to exit, let us do a little thinking along these lines, that we may be able to give relief more effectively and have disease more fully under our control.

Scientific Massage

Massage is known to be one of the oldest accepted methods in the healing art to be used by man in his age-old attempt to relieve pain and suffering. It had its beginning before the days of recorded history, some five thousand years ago. Massage was mentioned three hundred and eighty years before the time of Christ.

In 1783 Dr. Francis Holm speaks of friction.

In 1871 George Taylor, M.D., of New York City wrote a book of eight hundred pages on massage and its effect on the circulatory system.

No one will deny that scientific massage can be used to relieve many an ache or pain, by removing obstruction and freeing the circulation, thus giving tone to nerve and muscle tissue.

In ancient Greece, Hippocrates, the father of medicine, realized its value and taught it to his pupils.

It is recognized by men of science today for its remarkable healing power.

It is a therapeutic measure generally accepted and widely used.

We can then be led to believe that through perfect circulation a healthy body will make its own medicine and build up a chemical resistance to destructive disease.

Efficiency

Let me offer an important suggestion to increase your efficiency and save valuable time and energy when giving a Reflexology treatment—it is to be *more specific* than I find the average operator inclined to be.

Avoid any discussion of politics or current events with your patient. Such talk would prevent your efficiency from being on the alert and ready to determine from his expression at what moment you are in *direct contact* with these tiny nerve reflexes. His expression and reaction, as you contact these pain impulses, are an accurate guide in locating the point of congestion to be worked out by this form of foot Reflexology.

Now you are safe in assuring him that over a period of not too long a time this tenderness will disappear. When he asks *how long?* you should explain that it will depend on how long the congestion has been allowed to accumulate and how long these areas have been failing to contract and relax as nature intended they should.

CONCENTRATION

Most of your work may be done in places where you will encounter distractions. However, if you wish to be most efficient, learn to concentrate on what you are doing, regardless of your patient's persistent effort to tell you his symptoms or experiences with doctors and nurses during some previous operation.

Self-concentration is very necessary to enable you to know *just when* to turn from one affected or tender reflex to another, at the *proper time,* when it seems that a sufficient amount of pressure has been applied to the tender area.

Neglect of self-concentration will cause you to fail in applying the specific measures necessary for desired results.

Illustration of Technique

You have heard it said, "There is only one disease, physical or mental, and its name is congestion."

Let us hope that those who favor progressive methods of professional advancement will maintain an open mind and investigate the INGHAM COMPRESSION METHOD OF REFLEXOLOGY.

UNIQUE, BUT MOST EFFECTIVE

It is unique, but most effective, when scientifically applied as herein outlined:

It is the use of the thumb, such as you would use with the right thumb if trying to pulverize a few grains of granulated sugar in the palm of your left hand.

It is not just a steady pressure, but a slow creeping and slight pulling back movement, such as would be effective in dealing with a crystalline deposit formation for the purpose of breaking up or pulverizing the granules in the artery and nerve terminals in the feet.

Successful Practitioner

The successful practitioner will hold his attention under strict control of his findings. He will concentrate his attention on the intensity of pressure each patient can endure.

Let the patient know you are not trying to inflict unnecessary pain or discomfort. He may be inclined to refer to it as a form of torture treatment, as many do. Strange to say, however, instinct seems to convince patients that the tenderness you have located indicates an abnormal condition. When you explain what you are trying to do, that you are endeavoring to break up the congestion, giving them a certain amount of information as to the principles of your method, they will continue under your care until such tenderness has been worked out, if they wish to recover.

SKEPTICISM

They may express their disbelief that this tenderness could ever be worked out with Reflexology therapy. One man said to me, in answer to an assertion to this effect. "Well, maybe you are right; I am not accustomed to calling a lady a liar." I replied, "It has been done for others and unless you are an exception to the general rule, why not in your particular case?"

I was happily surprised, for in his case it really worked out quicker than usual. He was saved from an operation for prostate trouble, for which arrangements had already been made, even the date had been set. I believe he visited my office not more than eight to ten times and his troubles were over and he no longer had to get up every hour during the night to urinate.

TIME FOR RESULTS IMPOSSIBLE TO PREDICT

It is impossible to answer the question as to *how long* or *how many* treatments will be required to work out the tenderness.

I find it depends on how much vitality the patient may have and his ability to respond in carrying off that potent poison being thrown into the blood stream by this form of Reflexology. Again, it will depend on how long the congestion has been present. A chronic case will require a longer period for complete recovery, while an acute case may show improvement almost immediately.

Those who have been studying human history will acknowledge that man has not learned all there is to know on any given subject and probably never will. Knowledge, like time and space, seems to be infinity, and to feel that the saturation point has been reached is a grave danger.

Don't Be Hasty

Let us not be hasty in concluding that a theory is wrong simply because the facts are not proven conclusively to our personal way of thinking.

Generally speaking, it is safe to assume that not all physicians who are trained in medicine are always equally well trained in the mechanical treatment of disease. This situation automatically brings forth two different opinions. Both may be right, which tends to prove that the functions of the body and its various mechanisms are not altogether understood, with still a great deal remaining to be proven as fact.

As time passes and we become more proficient, we are better able to prove conclusively the value of reflex therapy to our esteemed medical colleagues. With history repeating itself, we are reminded that the science of medicine has often shown that what was once considered theory later became the accepted practice.

When Galileo expounded his belief that the world was round, he was nearly crucified. On his aged knees he was forced to retract his words and agree that the world was flat.

When Columbus started off to the West to find the East he could only engage a very few to sail with him who believed in his fantastic mission. Pasteur, Edison, Bell and Fulton all were denounced, challenged and ignored until their contributions to science could no longer be denied.

"What if wise men as far back as Ptolemy
   Thought that the earth, like an orange, was round;
None of them ever said, "Come along, follow me,
   Sail to the West and the East will be found."

Easy To Determine

It is easy to determine the location of each nerve impulse when you are familiar with the principle that the body can be divided into ten zones. This is known as THE INGHAM COMPRESSION METHOD OF REFLEXOLOGY, formerly referred to as ZONE THERAPY, or COMPRESSION MASSAGE.

When this fact of existing zone areas in the body was heretofore referred to as ZONE THERAPY, it was associated with a pressure method, used to desensitize or inhibit pain. This can definitely be used to some advantage where that is the object one wishes to attain. I would in no way want to discount its value for the purpose.

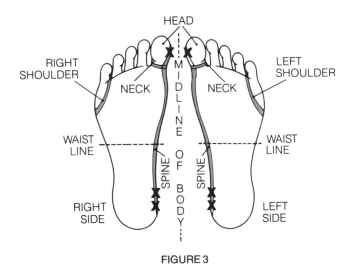

FIGURE 3

Here, however, we are dealing with the principle of ZONE THERAPY which tells the story in no uncertain terms as to where we may look for a definite reflex area in the feet which we wish to contact by this particular INGHAM COMPRESSION METHOD OF RELEXOLOGY. This method relaxes excessive nervous tension and breaks up the congestion we know to exist when there is any degree of tenderness in the areas at the nerve endings.

The function of pain is to indicate lowered vitality; therefore, pain is nature's way of telling us that trouble is at hand.

Pain

Pain is a protective mechanism of the body, an unpleasant reaction to massive stimulation of the sensory nerves calling attention to derangement of function disease or injury to a part as defined by *"Taber's Cyclopedic Medical Dictionary."* Thus pain in the reflexes as we discover them with this particular technique is not an enemy but an ally, an aid as an indication of where disease is to be found, calling our attention to some impaired function as the result of this congestion in the fine hair-like capillary system where nature is endeavoring to make that important transfer of the circulation from the arteries to the veins.

17

Reactions to be Expected

You may be surprised many times at the various types and forms of reaction which constitute the healing crisis following this form of reflex work. Keep in mind the process being carried on by nature and just what is being done when you apply this scientific technique to the tender reflexes in the feet.

Remember, tenderness means congestion, which indicates the existence of a potent poison at those particular terminals. When, through your work, this congestion has been broken up, nature has been called upon, by means of the circulatory system, to carry this potent poison to the organs of elimination, such as the liver, kidneys, lungs, skin, etc. If these are dormant in any way from an already existing toxic condition, you can well imagine the various forms of protest which follow when a new supply of this potent poison is set free and broken up for disposal.

IMPOSSIBLE TO PREDICT

It is impossible to predict in just what way or what form this reaction will manifest itself. Every individual, with varying tendencies, is a law unto himself. We do know we are relaxing a certain degree of nervous tension which aids in stimulating the circulation of the blood. This in turn increases the vitality so nature can throw off the poisons within.

I have seen it happen many times where, following the above procedure, the bowels have been caused to move twelve to fifteen times within twenty-four hours, without the slightest discomfort, such as would be experienced in a case of diarrhea. Just a manifestation of nature to the front to do her duty.

Now you can understand why I so strongly recommend that it is better not to give these treatments more often than twice a week. This applies especially in extreme cases where a great deal of poison is to be released, thus allowing nature a chance for her repair work.

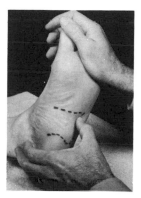

FIGURE 4
Position of Working the Reflex to the Colon.

No human being can heal our maladies, but we can help nature to renew our strength and fortitude to resist and correct the abnormalities that may afflict us. Thank God, healing does not wholly depend upon our faith in any particular method. It does help to know that others under similar conditions have been relieved by these natural means of assisting nature.

It is well to make faith the main spring of our life, keeping in mind the Biblical teaching that "Faith without works is dead." Thus it is the application of this work, this scientific method, applied to the nerve reflexes in the feet, combined with out knowledge and faith in its promises, that aids in prolonging life and useful activity.

Transgression against the laws of nature is the root of our afflictions.

Amount of Time

We have found that twenty to thirty minutes' time at the most, and this equally divided among the various tender areas of both feet, is long enough to spend with the average patient.

If the operator has been trained in our special technique for readily finding these reflexes, then the same work can be accomplished satisfactorily in half that length of time.

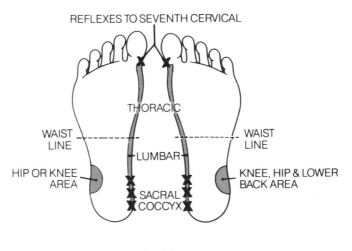

FIGURE 5

It will not be unusual for the patient to describe his feelings during the reactionary period somewhat to this effect, "I felt so bad I couldn't feel any worse, so I had to get better." This will happen, most likely, after the first, second or third treatment, depending to a great extent on the vitality of the patient to respond, after which time he will feel a definite improvement and an added degree of relief from each succeeding visit.

Osteopathic Concept

A spinal lesion means an abnormal pull on muscle tissue. If we can release the excessive tension by contacting a specific reflex in the feet, we are helping to bring about a correction of that spinal lesion. This occurs when nature decides to do so on her own, made possible by the added relaxation from our reflex work, or whether the aid of a skilled physician in that line has been called upon to hasten the recovery.

It has been my privilege to work in conjunction with those skilled in the osteopathic and chiropractic profession. Here, in connection with our research work, we have proved beyond all doubt that the INGHAM COMPRESSION METHOD OF REFLEXOLOGY applied to the spinal reflexes in the feet was an invaluable aid in producing added relaxation prior to any corrective measure, besides making the work of the practitioner more lasting in its effect.

It is the results we accomplish that we have to depend upon for continued success.

Can we deny the fact set forth by our osteopathic or chiropractic physicians that the secret of a greater part of our physical well-being lies in the condition of our spine?

The vertebra of the spine should be well separated from one another by cushions of firm cartilage in order to allow an unrestricted flow of blood and nerve supply to the various organs of our body.

If any degree of tenderness is found in those reflexes in that part of the foot relative to the spine, then by applying this form of compression technique to that area you will relax the muscle tension surrounding that vertebra. This tension may be retarding or preventing the correction of the abnormal condition, either through the natural movements of our body, which has been known to happen when the muscles were sufficiently relaxed, or by the mechanical skill of adjusting by one trained in that particular field.

. A muscle under strain is on its way to death and decay. A muscle carrying a load beyond its normal capacity by undue strain from some abnormal lesion tends to crystallize and lose its elasticity. Then what can we expect might follow, since disease is the product of strain. Any subluxation will intensify distortion. Obstruction to normal function is tension stress.

If we work in harmony with nature, we get results in spite of the wide gaps that still exist in our research work.

Coccyx Reflex

Following is a suggestion as to where we find it possible to relieve tension in that coccyx area so often found following an injury as the result of a fall which only a few have escaped. Since this area is the extreme end of the spinal column, we can readily understand why it could affect or distort the normal function of various organs and areas of the body. On page 20, Figure 5, of this section you will note the reflex area marked "Lumbar," following this down to the extreme end will be that of the coccyx. When this shows any degree of tenderness, work it out and you will be amazed many times at the results that will follow.

An Open Mind

May we retain an open and receptive mind for aid or suggestions in the scientific explanation of the relation of these nerve reflexes and their direct association with the tissues involved.

It seems reasonable to believe that the accumulation of the by-products of metabolism, the digestion and absorption of food, may cause deposits to form at the nerve reflexes. These deposits interfere with the normal nerve impulses so as to act as a resistance, much in the same manner as a transformer cuts down the current in a power line to a given point.

In the case of the transformer, of course, it is done for improvement, while in our consideration it proves to be a detrimental factor. In any event, to those of us who have had sufficient experience with this work, we know it definitely produces results.

I would like to see more research work done on this subject and would be glad to hear from anyone as to new developments in this field.

A SPIRIT OF MEEKNESS

Let us manifest a spirit of meekness and admit that we are only an instrument for good in the healing art. When a patient comes to us for help, if the condition is one that can be relieved by this reflex method, more power to us if we are sufficiently proficient to administer what is needed for his particular case.

Remember, no one method is complete in itself for the relief of every patient. When an adjustment of some vertebra is necessary to relieve a particular nerve impingement, the patient should be given the attention of a physician skilled in that particular art of healing. If surgery is required, as we all know to be true in some cases, the patient should have the services of a surgeon.

We have never seen a nerve impulse, but we know it exists. Any interference will lessen the speed of that impulse. Nerve tissue is more sensitive than any other tissue of the body.

No single science approaches completeness. A little knowledge here and a little there applied to whatever method you may already be using to help suffering humanity may prove a priceless asset to your success.

May I urge you to remember, "If at first you don't succeed, try, try again." Do not discredit the method because you do not get immediate results, any more than you would expect to play successfully on the piano without first having a knowledge of the proper chords and where and how to place the thumbs and fingers on the respective keys to produce the harmony desired.

Personality

Did you ever stop to consider what an important influence our glands have on the type and quality of our personality?

We are constantly throwing out a certain amount and quality of vibration which shows the type of our personality. We all want to be the possessor of a pleasing personality, but to have this we must look well to the functioning of our ductless glands, known as endocrine glands.

The voluntary vibrations are said to proceed from the brain through what we see with our eyes and say with our vocal cords, etc. The emotional phase of our involuntary vibrations, however, is controlled largely by the endocrine glands.

How important then that we pay attention and adopt any method which will help maintain a healthy condition of these important glands of our body, if we want to have a pleasing personality, throwing out vibrations that will attract better health. As one of the old Hermetic writers has said, "He who understands the principle of vibrations has grasped the sceptre of power."

The Chinese claim that the magnetic forces come through the soles of the feet, which act as a receiving station.

Prof. Rudolf Virchow, Master Physician of the World says, "The eternal fires within you still glows, even to the bottom of your soles."

Emotions

Our emotions constitute the main spring of life, the driving force for good or ill effects. We cannot separate the power of emotions from that of mind and thought. This explains why the number of victims suffering from stomach ulcer has been known to go up or down with the stock market quotations. This tells the story of some improper glandular balance, undoubtedly caused by excessive nervous tension.

To correct an unbalanced emotional condition, let us see if one particular gland may be affected more than another.

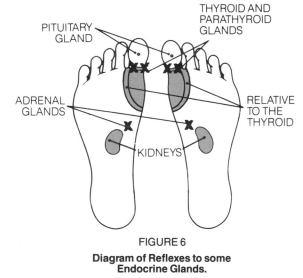

FIGURE 6

Diagram of Reflexes to some Endocrine Glands.

We will contact the specific reflex to each particular gland to see which one shows the greatest degree of tenderness.

Although the glands function so nearly in unison, yet when we thoroughly understand WHAT STORIES THE FEET CAN TELL, we know from the location of the greatest degree of tenderness which gland is failing primarily in its ability to contract and relax as nature intended it should to prevent a crystalline deposit formation from accumulating at its own particular reflex area.

With this discovery in mind, get busy and work out the congestion responsible for this tenderness so each gland can again perform its own particular duty by furnishing the proper hormone secretion required by nature for a healthy mind and body. Your patient will then be able to reason normally and the added strain of useless emotions, such as fear and worry, will disappear.

There is a legitimate concern resulting from a healthy mind that is not wasteful fear, but worry resulting from an abnormal glandular system is carrying tomorrow's load on today's haul, an added strain of useless emotions.

Regret is akin to worry. There may be pages in our life's history we wish we had not written. Is this not a fact with us all? To regret some past experience in our life for which we can still make amends is all well and good. Our regret then becomes a God-given emotional disturbance and we can shut the door on yesterday's decision and look to this day, for it is life.

Look To This Day

Look to this day!
For it is life, the very life of life.
In its brief course lie all the verities
    and realities of your existence:
The bliss of growth;
The glory of action;
The splendor of beauty;
For yesterday is already a dream,
    and tomorrow is only a vision;
But today, well lived, makes every
    yesterday
A dream of happiness, and every
    tomorrow a vision of hope.
Look well, therefore, to this day!
Such the salutation of the dawn!

—From the Sanskrit

The Power of Thought

What fortifies the mind under strain more than habitual cheerfulness? The power of this and its effect upon the human body cannot be emphasized too strongly. It is comparable to a healthy balance in your account.

Everything about this bodily machine in health is functioning according to God's great laws of nature, and given its greatest boost when we are cheerful and happy.

Who can offer an adequate substitute for a happy and healthy home life? The power of thought can make us live or die. Yes, the power of our thoughts can make us live a happy and healthy life, or fill our body with poison, resulting in pain and disease.

Let us will ourselves to live to be ninety or one hundred years old, not simply saying the words, but meaning them and believing it can be done.

We can really invite disaster by our negative fears and thoughts and bring about many a serious condition from the effect these negative thoughts will have on the functioning of our glands, changing the normal metabolic balance.

Fear is a poison that can affect every part of the human organism.

Influence of Worry

Worry is derived from a Saxon word that means to choke. This fits in with the idea we are trying to convey that one can choke off a portion of the normal blood supply to various parts of the body by refusing to stop needless worry.

We are told by some authorities that circulation follows attention. With this in mind a good way to help many unpleasant conditions would be to practice the art of forgetting. A man is what he forgets. The essence of genius is to know what to forget.

Referring to the Bible we find the same thought expressed by the Apostle Paul in his Epistle to the Philippians, chapter 3, verses 13 to 15, where he says, "But one thing I do, forgetting those things which are behind, and reaching forth unto those things which are before, I press toward the mark for the prize of the high calling of God in Christ Jesus. Let us therefore, as many as be perfect, be thus minded."

How important then for us to realize that if one is full of fear and worry he becomes tense and unable to relax. The circulation becomes partially choked in certain areas, the tiny capillaries in the feet become choked with a crystalline deposit formation, interfering with the circulation and the normal transference of the blood from the arteries to the veins which must take place at those terminals. The result of this is the tenderness we encounter when we contact these special reflexes in the feet.

ARE WE ONLY HALF ALIVE?

As long as we are alive we have to live. Do we care to be just half alive, or shall we conquer our fears and be among those who are up and doing and alive to their finger tips?

How many are sick because they fail to organize their emotions, fail to acknowledge the law of God and nature that governs the human body, a most intricate machine, worthy of the best knowledge and effort we can put forth to keep it in perfect working order.

LIMITATION AND FEAR

Our only limitation in the achievements of tomorrow will be our fears of today. Regardless of what method we use in an effort to correct an abnormal physical condition, if the above limitation exists, our success will be limited.

It is well to study the mental attitude of your patient to determine the degree of progress you may hope to attain. Where fear and anxiety are affecting the functioning of the glands it will take longer to get results. Often this can be traced primarily to a condition where childhood environment plays an important part.

Many times it is advisable to discuss this possibility with your patient, which may help him in changing his mental attitude and have a relaxing effect on the nervous system.

NO SET TIME FOR A DEFINITE IMPROVEMENT

The fact that anxiety is becoming more and more a common factor lying behind many cases of poor health gives rise to the fact that it is impossible to have a set rule as to how soon we will meet with a definite improvement.

Should failure attend your efforts, do not condemn the reflex work, for it is not a form of magic attended by some hocus-pocus words or movements. Instead it is a scientific form of contacting the nerve impulses in the feet relative to the various organs of the body, and a method of stimulating the glands of internal secretion.

I entreat you to try this INGHAM COMPRESSION METHOD OF REFLEXOLOGY when called upon to help anyone in need of relaxation.

Learn the correct technique for contacting these various reflexes where *any degree* of tenderness can be found, and then work it out. It cannot be done over night. Let me say again, the length of time required for this will depend on how long that congestion has existed and how nearly you have mastered the art of finding the tender reflexes to be worked out.

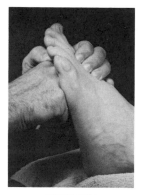

FIGURE 7

**Position for loosening muscles
of the shoulder and neck.**

Anger

Anger produces poison, so do not generate more indignation than you have the capacity to control.

Do not let the wild forces of your nature run loose and fill the body with poison from anger that is not under your emotional control.

Anger produces more poison than fear.

Anger misdirected becomes a destructive element.

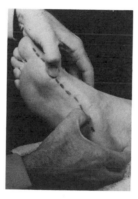

FIGURE 8
Position for Working the Reflexes
to the Spine (both feet).

Again your attention is called to the wise words in the Bible, Proverbs, chapter 16, verse 32: "He that is slow to anger is better than the mighty; and he that ruleth his spirit than he that taketh a city."

Hormones

Much is being written at the present time regarding the hormones and their importance to our well-being.

We use the term hormone to describe a chemical substance produced by the various endocrine glands of our body.

When speaking of hormones we are calling your attention to a chemical substance, such as that produced by one gland and then transported to some other gland or organ of the body to produce a specific effect.

Since the pituitary gland governs the functioning of the other glands, then it is the chemical produced by the anterior lobe of the pituitary gland, referred to as hormones, that sends out a certain substance which has power to influence the adrenal glands.

The hormone produced by this anterior lobe acts not only on the adrenal glands, but also on the ovaries. It plays an important part in pregnancy and is a causative agent in normal menstruation. The hormone produced by the posterior lobe of the pituitary gland acts more as a regulator and is an important substance for normal heart muscles, a normal heart beat, and a most necessary substance for dilating the arteries.

It is a hormone, chemical substance, from the anterior lobe of the pituitary gland that blends with the insulin to regulate carbohydrate metabolism, the digestion and absorption of starches and sugars. Now you can understand why I emphatically recommend that you work on the reflexes to the pituitary gland when dealing with any case of diabetes. Read page 38 in my book, *"Stories The Feet Can Tell."*

IMPOSSIBLE TO DIFFERENTIATE

It is impossible to differentiate between these two lobes from a reflex angle, since the pituitary gland is so small, but I say, again and again, *find* the tender reflex and work it out, whether it is the anterior or posterior lobe at fault. You are working to create the normal functioning of this master gland.

> If you're feeling out of kilter,
> Don't know why or what about,
> Let your feet reveal the answer,
> Find the sore spot, work it out.

Do not be disturbed if you are uncertain as to the exact meaning of the story being told; just keep in mind that *every* tender reflex tells its own story. Whether you can read that story accurately at first matters very little. It will not prevent you from getting results. You are going to find the sore spot and work it out, regardless of your ability to know the answer.

A POINT TO REMEMBER

It is well to remind you that when doing this form of reflex work you are only applying a particular form of compression technique to the reflexes in the feet. You are not diagnosing. You are not prescribing. You are in no way practicing medicine, but simply using a reflex method to help relieve nerve tension to stimulate the circulation so nature can restore the normal functioning of the various glands and organs of the body.

Relationship of Glands

It is important to gain all the knowledge we can of the vast variety of results that come from derangements of the glandular system and its apparently eccentric members.

I learned a great deal from a most instructive book I secured from the library recently, entitled, *"What We Are And Why"* by Laurence H. Mayers, M.D., Professor of Medical research in the Medical School of Western University. It deals with his discoveries on subjects like these, "What Are The Sources Of Behavior?" and "Why Do We Grow Tall Or Fat, Or Criminal Or Moral?"

So far as Dr. Mayers has gone, the causes lie in functioning of the endocrine glands that are distributed throughout our body. He has taken photographs of people in series, at ten years old, twenty, thirty, forty, to show how the child of ten, who because he has had the mumps, thus disturbing the normal functioning of these glands, became abnormal, enormously tall, enormously fat, or unbalanced morally. He also tells us that the disturbance of one gland may cause functional derangement of another that will show only in the structure of the bone, a system of relationship only partially understood.

As I have said before, and repeat again, if the reflex to any one gland is tender, try that of the other glands also, to be sure you are reaching the *real cause* of your patient's disturbance.

If you are treating a case diagnosed as only nerves, remember what Dr. Mayers has been telling us that the thyroid hormone contains iodine, which is indispensable to life and sanity, and that each of us is removed from idiocy by just about two milligrams of iodine, supplied daily by the thyroid gland.

Can A Gland be Removed by Surgery?

Some of these important glands can be partially removed and yet the remaining portion of that gland induced to increase its activity to supply what the body requires for nearly normal functioning.

Where no surgery has been applied, we can expect results more quickly. However despite any operation that may have preceded your work, I feel confident that no harm could ensue, for with this method you are simply normalizing the condition, helping nature to function more efficiently.

We must admit that without glands in our body we would fail to exist. Then we can see how much depends upon our knowledge of such important organs of the body and that we should do everything in our power to maintain perfect harmony in the performance of their duty.

We find that fear, worry, grief and disappointment are direct enemies of the well-being of these glands. Many times these enemies are hard to eradicate until considerable harm has been done by their emotional disturbance. If we can strengthen these glands by releasing the excessive tension and nourish them with a better blood supply, they will again be able to function normally, giving the patient a proper outlook on life.

Any problem is met and solved more satisfactorily if we meet it face to face with a healthy mind and body. Remember, it is up to us, to a great extent, in what manner we meet the conflicts that beset our pathways.

Glandular Deficiency

I often feel that I would like to specialize in helping those who suffer from some glandular deficiency, especially if we can prove the cause is not altogether a mental attitude.

Those who have been using this corrective method successfully agree with me implicitly that the secret of our success in relieving such a variety of abnormal conditions is due to the relaxation produced by the use of this particular technique, known as the INGHAM COMPRESSION METHOD OF REFLEXOLOGY.

This method, applied to the reflexes in the feet, not only breaks up the congestion of those terminals, but definitely relaxes the hypertension responsible for so many ills of the present day.

Thus it is reasonable to believe that with this knowledge at hand you will obtain results in practically any condition which can be helped by relaxing nerve tension, increasing the circulation and the vitality so that nature will have the power to throw off the accumulated poisons.

Solar Plexus

Our next consideration will be the solar plexus, a center of nerve influence, a great network of nerves, giving off nerves to all parts of the abdominal cavity, sometimes called the abdominal brain.

It is situated behind the stomach and in front of the diaphragm.

It distributes fine thread-like nerves under the name of plexuses, which accompany all the branches from the front of the abdominal aorta, the part of the aorta below the diaphragm, as well as the supra-renal (adrenal) glands.

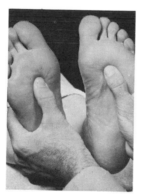

FIGURE 9
Position for Relieving Tension Through the Solar Plexus.

With the thumb of your right hand contact the solar plexus reflex on the left foot of your patient. Then place the thumb of your left hand on the reflex on the right foot. Now apply a steady pressure to both feet at the same time, increasing the pressure while the patient inhales deeply; then release it gradually while he exhales. Repeat this, according to rhythm six or eight times. You will be likely to notice an expression of relaxation almost immediately.

DIAPHRAGM

With the method outlined above you will definitely affect the diaphragm which, as a large muscle, serves as a partition, a muscular wall which separates the thorax from the abdomen.

Can you imagine the importance of maintaining the normal elasticity of this muscle if we are to remain receptive to the life-giving forces surrounding us through which the act of restoration is constantly being carried on?

Every time a muscle contracts or has a squeezing effect on the blood vessels, especially the veins, thus aiding the circulatory system.

The more we maintain the elasticity of this diaphragm muscle the more easily we will be able to inhale oxygen, the life giving force, a necessary element that helps to burn up the toxic poison in our system.

Pituitary Gland

I will endeavor to explain in this chapter the marvelous results that can be produced by compression technique applied to the reflex area leading to the pituitary gland. This reflex is found in the center of the ball of each big toe. See Fig. 6 Pg. 26.

This master gland is located at the base of the brain. Hence we must remember that any congestion in the back of the neck or surrounding area will definitly retard the blood supply and interfere with the normal functioning of this important gland. This condition would not exist if the gland were being supplied with the perfect circulation nature intended it to have.

The pituitary gland cannot be deprived of its life-giving forces, through hypertension or injury, without disastrous results. This often causes inability to reason normally. Have we not all seen emotional disturbances that could be traced to nervous tension which had impeded the blood supply to this gland?

Here we have the primary cause of many a nervous breakdown.

This poison or debris in the blood stream may be likened to a plumbing system where the drain pipes require the attention of a plumber. He takes the rubber cup with a handle, fills the sink with water, covering the outlet, and starts pulsating, creating a terrific intermittent pressure, freeing the drain of all obstructions. The water begins to flow and the circulation is restored from the use of this rubber pump.

Thus we have shown how important is this method of compression technique, if it can relieve nervous tension sufficiently to create a renewed amount of circulation, by setting up a pulsating system which loosens any crystalline formation of residue from the blood stream, putting it into suspension where eventually it can be eliminated.

Just as stepping on a lawn hose lessens the pressure and supply of water, pressure on nerves will slow down the body functions. Normal nerve force depends upon normal circulation.

CASE HISTORY

Let me relate an interesting experience I had not long ago. Mr. D., a high school teacher for thirty years, became so nervous and exhausted after the school term that he felt he was ready to die. He believed he was seriously ill. He visited one specialist after another, who made numerous tests, thorough examinations, X-rays, etc. None had been successful in finding any serious ailments. His mental attitude was condemnation for them all. He could not sleep and told me he walked the floor nights with only two things in mind—murder and suicide.

I soon had his feet in my hands and found WHAT STORIES THEY COULD BE MADE TO TELL. Just as I expected, the physicians' diagnoses were correct. No physical ailment existed, except the condition of his nerves.

With the corner of my thumb, I pressed deeply into the ball of each big toe, the reflex to the pituitary gland. He said it felt as if it were being pierced with a piece of broken glass. The sides of each big toe were tender, proving he had a great deal of congestion in the back of his neck. This prevented the proper circulation to his brain, cutting off normal nerve impulses to this important area governing his nervous system.

I then proceeded to the gland reflexes described more fully in my book "STORIES THE FEET CAN TELL." However, there was only a slight tenderness to be found in these reflexes, such as the thyroid, located under the root of the big toe; the adrenal, above the kidney reflex in the center of the foot; and the prostate, under and just below the ankle bone. His mental attitude had caused him to worry and imagine that he had serious ailments. See Fig. 6, Pg. 26.

After about ten to fifteen minutes of compression technique applied deeply to these various reflexes intermittently, the pain gradually lessened. By this time he began to feel relaxed. That night he slept normally several hours without a sedative. Three days later I saw him again. The treatment was not repeated sooner, as nature had to adjust gradually to the relaxation brought about by this work and the newly added supply of secretion from these glands now being sent into the blood stream.

In two to three weeks the tenderness had disappeared and he was now able to sleep at night. He could carry on a conversation normally. It was encouraging to see him take an entirely new attitude toward life. Feeling so much better after taking a few treatments, he would try to find the tender places and work them himself. I encouraged him to do so, as I had explained to him the method I was using and how accurate it was in determining the cause of his nervous tension. He stopped worrying and when school started he was in the pink of condition and ready to return to his teaching.

Insomnia

I have had excellent results in cases of insomnia by applying the INGHAM COMPRESSION METHOD OF REFLEXOLOGY to the reflexes leading to the pituitary gland.

We all know what disastrous results can follow persistent insomnia. Let me ask you here to follow closely what I am giving you for releasing nervous tension caused by a defective functioning of the pituitary gland.

Disturbed nerve control, worry or any distressing factor, have influence in causing insomnia. The patient who is unable to sleep, due to the hypertension built up from an emotional disturbance will, during those wakeful hours when the imagination runs rampant, let a most absurd thought take on the form of reality.

The heart action will increase, blood pressure go up, sending an abnormal supply of glandular (hormone) secretion into the blood stream, changing the normal chemistry of the body. Can you see why six and one-half million sleeping pills will be taken tonight?

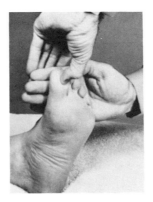

FIGURE 10

**Position for Working the Reflex
to the Pituitary Gland.**

With the picture in mind of the location of the reflexes to the back of the neck you will deeply work the inside and outside edge of each big toe to relieve congestion in the area supplying blood to the pituitary gland.

Roll the corner of your thumb, with a deep hooking movement, into the center of the ball of each big toe, aiming for a pinpoint area.

For a specific direct contact with the reflexes to the pituitary gland see Fig. 10.

Remember, the reflex to the pituitary gland is only the size of a pin point and unless you make that particular specific contact with the corner of your thumb you will fail to get the results you are seeking to obtain.

Acromegaly

This is an abnormal development, chiefly of the bones of the face and extremities, associated with disease of the pituitary and thyroid glands.

I could write volumes on the variety of cases I have been able to help simply by correcting the cause of a sick pituitary gland that has been robbed of its normal blood supply.

Since the pituitary gland is considered the master of the glandular system, we can expect help from this source for a great number of ailments. It is responsible not only for the growth of our giants, but the midget can blame that tiny gland for his difference in height.

The medical profession has recently come to the conclusion that a rare condition known as acromegaly is caused by an overactive pituitary gland, where the lips, face, hands and feet take on an abnormal appearance by growing out of proportion to almost double the normal size.

The facial expression changes. The face becomes massive. The tongue, lips and nose are thickened until one who may have been attractive even goodlooking, will take on the expression and appearance of an ape.

A pitiful condition is this disease known as acromegaly. It can transform the fair and beautiful to ugliness, the graceful to awkwardness, the strong to weakness, and the active to sluggishness.

Acromegaly may be preceded by severe headaches, as I found to be the case with a patient I recently examined. The pituitary gland reflex was extremely tender. His home being in a distant city, I was unable to give him my reflex work, which I am confident would have given better results than the heavy X-ray treatments he resorted to for relief.

Physicians tell us acromegaly is often accompanied by some alternation of the genitals (sex glands), and likely the adrenals.

Again I want to remind you that if you find a tender reflex to any one of these important glands, work it out, for who knows what disastrous results you may be the means of intercepting.

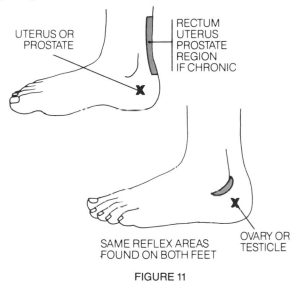

UTERUS OR
PROSTATE

RECTUM
UTERUS
PROSTATE
REGION
IF CHRONIC

SAME REFLEX AREAS
FOUND ON BOTH FEET

OVARY OR
TESTICLE

FIGURE 11

I have found the pituitary gland tender in so many cases that it is the first place I look to for trouble where any nerve or glandular condition is involved.

I cannot begin to estimate the amount of good that can be done by this reflex work. You, like myself, will often be amazed by the astonishing results you will obtain.

Prostate Gland

As we approach middle life we all experience disorders with the generative organs, which involve the prostate gland in the male and the ovaries in the female. It is well known that the ailments which befall humanity when these glands fail to function often produce a great deal of discomfort and inconvenience.

You will encounter frequently in the male an enlarged prostate gland, a condition causing the patient to urinate sometimes as often as every hour, day and night, and which may also be accompanied by considerable pain.

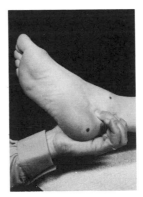

FIGURE 12
Location for Working the Reflex
to the Prostate Gland (Both Feet).

This condition will respond very rapidly if the INGHAM COMPRESSION METHOD OF REFLEXOLOGY is applied. Hold the heel of the right foot in the left hand, using the third finger to apply the technique half way between the anklebone and the point of the heel. See Fig,12. This should also be done on the left foot with the right hand in the same manner.

Your patient may cry out for mercy, so try not to be too severe. It is not necessary to cause too much pain at any one time. Explain to your patient that if the prostate gland were functioning as nature intended it should, there would be no pain, this particular reflex would not be tender, and there would be no formation of crystalline deposits or abnormal end products. However, when there is an abnormal condition of this gland working the specific reflex is necessary to break up the congestion in that area so it can be carried through the blood stream to the organs of elimination. As the tenderness begins to disappear, the patient will feel a marked improvement.

CASE HISTORY

I recall one extreme case brought to my office not long ago. Mr. T., was being called upon to urinate every hour, day and night. This was accompanied by such extreme pain he felt the only relief for him was an operation. Before his first treatment was completed he went into the bathroom and returned with tears in his eyes, saying, "You have really done something for me. It doesn't seem possible, but for the first time in three months I have urinated without pain and was able to eliminate a normal amount instead of only a few drops."

I continued to apply this reflex method faithfully, not more often than twice a week, and when he returned to his physician for examination he was amazed to be told that the enlarged gland had definitely decreased in size, and without an operation. He continued to improve as the tenderness worked out until he could go to bed and sleep all night.

When dealing with any abnormal prostate condition, remember, a chronic case will show a tenderness over a larger area up on the inside part of the leg but the most important point of contact will be a pinpoint area found half way between the ankle bone and edge of the heel. This will be found tender when a condition is still in the acute stage.

I have recieved a great many letters from those using this compression method of Refexology, telling of cases very much like this which they had been able to relieve. Just as a gland has grown into an abnormal condition, through nervous tension and the lack of proper circulation, so will it return to normal when the cause has been corrected.

Let us strive to increase our knowledge of any new discovery that may help suffering humanity. Since it is a well known fact that no single method of healing provides complete care for all the ills of mankind.

Thyroid Gland

The thyroid gland, located on each side of the trachea (windpipe), has two lobes which are connected by an isthmus stretching across the front of the neck, the cavities of which are occupied by an iodine-containing material, the active principle of which keeps us in tune with our surroundings.

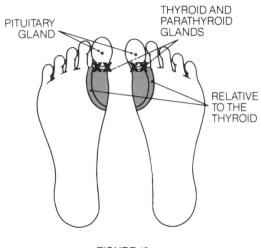

PITUITARY GLAND

THYROID AND PARATHYROID GLANDS

RELATIVE TO THE THYROID

FIGURE 13

The thyroid gland is closely related to other members of the endocrine system, any derangement of which may affect the other, especially the pituitary and adrenal glands.

The demands of the body are somewhat particular. An oversupply or a deficiency of hormone secretion from any one of these glands will be sure to cause an abnormal condition, sending one in search of a method of relief.

Thus we find a sound basis for the conclusion that normal functioning of the glands and harmony in their adjustment to each other is indispensable to a normal harmonious development.

SUBSTITUTE THERAPY

Much is being written from time to time regarding the substitution of glandular therapy, that of supplying the gland product by needle, temporarily providing relief, like ACTH, cortisone, insulin, etc.

But with this form of reflex work we are dealing with a stimulating gland therapy, that of causing each gland, by added stimulation, to produce its own normal hormone. Each gland, as it improves, will have an added influence on the wellbeing of the other glands.

Who would not prefer to have the functioning of his glands restored to normal so nature can produce her own glandular secretion?

It is this hormone secretion produced by the thyroid gland that calls upon the chemical laboratory of the body for fuel to supply energy. If this fuel supply is not forthcoming, we have a mentally heavy, dull personality, like those who have been styled as "born tired, inattentive, asleep at the switch."

It is believed that many criminals and inmates of mental institutions are the victims of a thyroid deficiency. If it has reached the stage where it is manifesting itself in the form of a simple goiter, we know there is a deficiency of iodine being produced, the absence of which is responsible for the enlargement, due to the accumulation of a jelly-like substance known as colloid.

DIFFERENT KINDS OF GOITER

We learn that several different kinds of goiter exist, each producing different effects, yet having one thing in common, a disorder of or a defect in the functioning of the thyroid gland.

By placing the finger lightly just below the Adam's

Apple you will be able to feel the thyroid gland, a vital agent in regulating weight, body activities, etc.

It is the hormones sent into the blood stream by the thyriod gland that we depend upon for normal metabolism. The first definition of metabolism in *"Sander's American Medical Dictionary"* is: "Tissue change, the sum of all the physical and chemical processes by which living organized substance is produced and maintained, and the transformation by which energy is made available for the uses of organism." (organic structure)

Now it is easy to understand what is meant when we are told that metabolism, a tissue change governed by the hormones supplied from the thyroid gland, is the burning, or the combustive quality necessary to eliminate the poisons. It is likened to the process where fuel releases heat to create steam to maintain respiration, a necessary medium to obtain oxygen to keep the fire going—circulation, muscle tone and glandular activity.

The hormone substance is very important for breaking down the waste products of the body, splitting up the uric acid which has become the end product of nitrogen, makeing possible its elimination through the kidneys.

53

Thus a deficiency in the functioning of the thyroid gland to produce a sufficient amount of thyroid hormones will result in a metabolism minus test, a deficiency in the fuel to combust or break up the poison in the system. This could be the starting point for obesity, overweight, etc., usually referred to as a hypothyroid case.

Instead of the usual form of treatment for this condition, which is that of supplying a thyroid substitute, would it not be more satisfactory if we knew how to apply this IN-GHAM COMPRESSION METHOD OF REFLEXOLOGY in a way that would stimulate the action of the thyroid gland and enable it to produce its own normal secretion according to nature's plan?

OVERACTIVE THYROID

When an overactive thyroid condition exists the symptoms will be the opposite. A very talkative person may be found, with shifting moods, hypersensitive, and one hard to cope with, although he may appear in good health, with eyes alert, lustrous hair and the skin warm and moist from excessive persiration.

This condition, known as hyperthyroidism, causes profound internal changes. It can bring on hypertension (high blood pressure) and a breakdown in the functioning of the kidneys.

There is no way to determine from the reflex angle which one of these two conditions exists. From the outward expression, when the eyes present a bulging appearance, it is quite evident the patient is suffering from hyperthyroidism. But regardless of what we are endeavoring to correct, whether you are dealing with hypothyroidism or hyperthyroidism, your work on these reflex areas of the feet will be to relax and normalize the excessive tension that may be responsible for either condition.

CASE HISTORY

An outstanding case I remember is that of a young lady, twenty-three years old, a school teacher, whose duties and responsibilities had brought about a complete nervous breakdown.

She was taken to the hospital for observation and confined to a padded cell. Her parents were acquainted with the work I was doing with this method and persuaded the physicians to let them bring her home with a trained nurse. A bedroom was equipped for this purpose, as every piece of furniture had to be removed except a box spring and mattress placed in a corner on the floor and one heavy oak office chair was all that remained since her strength seemed superhuman and she was determined to destroy everything.

I was told to remove my glasses before entering. I trusted the hand of Providence to protect me. The nurse opened the door and the patient stepped toward me and informed me at once that I would need a hair-do when she got through with me. I succeeded in diverting her attention by saying that since she could drive I had come to ask if she would go to Florida with me for the winter. I explained how nice it would be and what we could do, etc. She stood attentive and I explained at length that I had heard she could not sleep. I told her that if she would let me work on her feet, it would help her to sleep without having to take the hypos she so violently opposed.

Strange as it may seem, I soon had her feet in my hands. As I started to use the pressure on the pituitary gland reflex in the ball of the big toe, she made no protest, but talked constantly and incoherently. After I had been applying the pressure pretty steadily she stopped rambling long enough to say, "How about giving that toe a rest for awhile and trying the other one?" I ordered a pillow and blanket and for the first time in two weeks she went to sleep for five hours, without a sedative, the strongest form of which had been having little or no effect.

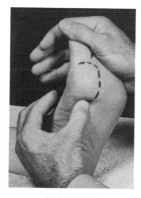

FIGURE 14
Position for Working the Reflex
to the Thyroid Gland (Both Feet).

The next day she was still violent and restless, even more so, as I had expected her to be, for I had worked on the reflex areas to the thyroid and adrenal glands, which were also somewhat tender. I knew the effect of what I had done would be to give the system a fresh supply of these glandular secretions to which it would have to adjust in various ways.

I waited six days. When I returned she was dressed and downstairs in the living room, still badly confused. As I opened the door she called out to me, "Why did you stay away so long?" She willingly let me do all I felt was necessary. After the third visit, five days later, she was brought to my home for her treatments. Five weeks later she was driving her own car. When the January term of school opened she was again teaching. The tenderness had completely disappeared and she has been fine ever since.

Ovaries

Many abnormal conditions of the ovaries may be caused by an abnormal thyroid, so where the reflex to either of these important glands is tender remember the close relationship of one to the other.

You will find where a congestion exists causing discomfort during the menstrual period, after you have contacted those reflexes according to the principles outlined herein, the natural functioning of those glands can be restored to normal.

Remember the connection between the thyroid and ovaries. Trouble in one area may affect the other, and vice versa.

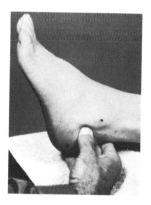

FIGURE 15
Position for Working the Reflex to the Ovaries.

Spleen

The spleen is also one of the important glands, located on the left side of the body above the waistline.

The spleen is said to absorb the particles of broken-down red corpuscles. It is a storehouse for additional iron needed by the blood.

The spleen also produces a substance which powerfully stimulates the intestinal peristalsis, acting upon both the small and large intestine.

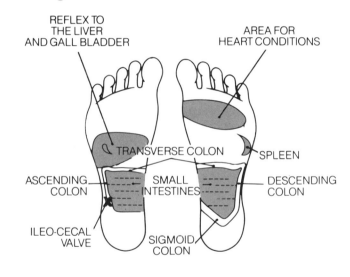

FIGURE 16

Thus, we do well to guard carefully the well-being of the liver and spleen, if we wish to maintain the benefit of their aid in preventing constipation, etc., through their ability to improve the movements of the alimentary canal.

Sympathetic Nerves

Our Sympathetic nervous reflex system sends its disorders to the surface of the body by way of the skin, etc., and may manifest itself in the form of a rash or hives. How often a condition of this kind will be diagnosed by the physician as just plain nerves.

Now what is responsible for this condition of *just plain nerves?* It may cause results that will be diagnosed as some form of allergy, which makes it possible for one person to be allergic to a certain food that will not affect another.

Are we to assume that an allergy just chose a special place to pester Mary Ann, and another place to annoy Susie Jane? Did Mary Ann have a deficiency in the thyroid hormone, resulting from an abnormal condition of the thyroid gland, which manifested itself differently from that of Susie Jane? Susie Jane's adrenal glands may have been below normal and failed to supply the kidneys with sufficient driving-force to eliminate the uric acid from the system sufficiently to prevent placing an abnormal load on the pores of the skin, for they play a very important part in carrying away the poisons of the system. Can you not see where any degree of nervous tension would affect the normal contraction and relaxation necessary for the pores to produce perspiration, which is their part in the system of elimination.

Thus when you find a dry scaly surface of the skin, look to the various gland reflexes to see which one shows the greatest degree of tenderness. This proves again WHAT STORIES THE FEET CAN BE MADE TO TELL as to which particular gland may be primarily at fault. Then proceed to break up the crystalline deposit formation which is causing that reflex to be tender and sensitive. This will relax the tension which has prevented these glands from doing their specific duty.

The results we obtain will reward us for our efforts and the know-how in bringing about the normal production of these hormones necessary for a healthy body and a healthy mind, a combination impossible to separate.

Headache

You will often be surprised at WHAT STORIES THE FEET CAN BE MADE TO TELL when it comes to determining the exact cause of the various types of headache we encounter. From a medical standpoint extensive tests are often necessary to rule out those caused by disease or those where a psychic factor may be involved. But with this form of reflex work we can determine from the area showing the greatest degree of tenderness the answer to our problem with very little effort.

If the headache can be forgotten when something important or interesting is to be accomplished, it is not likely to be organic and no particular tender reflex will be found.

If the ache originates at the back of the neck and proceeds up over the top of the head, it is doubtless the result of some emotional upset, the cause of which you will seek to find in the gland where the reflex shows the greatest degree of tenderness.

If the seventh or upper cervical region is at fault, work around the inside of each big toe, see Fig. 17, pg. 63. Then rotate them each way a few times. Then go into the center of the ball of each big toe to learn if it could be coming from an abnormal condition of the pituitary gland. Many a persistent common everyday headache will cease when you work deeply with the corner of your thumb the center and sides of each big toe see Fig. 10 pg. 44.

MIGRAINE

Your success in helping patients who suffer such excruciating pain as the result of migraine headache will depend to a great extent upon the specific cause in each particular case.

If you find that cause to be a definite physical or organic disorder which can be located and corrected by the INGHAM

COMPRESSION METHOD OF REFLEXOLOGY, your results will be phenomenal. But if instead, it is traced to a complex resulting from some unpleasant conditions in his home atmosphere, your patient will no doubt have to seek help from a psychiatrist or continue to live with the condition as a means of obtaining sympathy from friends and relatives.

It is hard to believe that anyone would, consciously or subconsciously, entertain such a painful condition for this purpose, but we are told that it is a fact, nevertheless, with a few who have a distorted mental attitude. This reminds me of the lady who said, "I have a lot of trouble, but I would not be without it. I find it such a comfort to tell other folks about."

OTHER CAUSES OF MIGRAINE

Many victims of migraine have reported that their headaches are preceded by symptoms of diarrhea, colitis, and an abnormal craving for food. With this in mind, we can see why elimination diets are found to give relief to some and why fasting is often temporarily beneficial to others.

In children it is advisable to look to the possibility of associating the migraine headache with some form of gastro-intestinal disturbance.

It is being brought to our attention at the present time by reliable medical authority that they believe migraine to be an edema of the brain tissue following an allergic response. Therefore, if migraine is not a disease, it, too, must be only a symptom.

When reading articles of late on allergies, etc., I have noticed how often when speaking of hives and eczema in children it will be linked to a further discussion of epilepsy and migraine. These are associated with severe gastro-intestinal conditions, emphasizing again the importance in such cases of the tiny ileocecal valve which is so important in the proper elimination of the mucous secretion from the small intestinal tract into the colon.

Now we can readily understand why people with migraine frequently complain of pains in the abdomen and of diarrhea which sometimes precede these headaches.

In 1777 the French word migraine appeared in our English literature, which described this particular affliction as a periodic one-sided headache, usually starting over one eye and spreading over the entire top of the head.

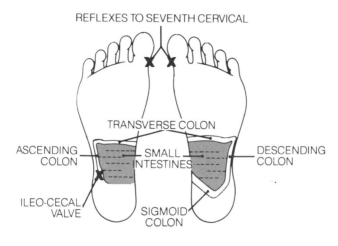

FIGURE 17

Arthritis

Let us consider our possibility for bringing relief to those who suffer from arthritis, neuritis, rheumatism, etc., all of which may have a common cause, depending to a great extent upon the chemical type of patient.

Much is being said and written at the present time of help being received by the use of ACTH, a hormone extracted from the pituitary and adrenal glands of certain animals. This is only claimed as helpful, a crutch, we will say, to lean upon to carry the patient over to a time when he will be able to produce from his own glandular system the necessary hormone element, the heat producing energy required by nature to break up and carry away the poison in our system.

If the governor, the pituitary gland, fails to issue certain orders to the adrenal glands, causing them to become confused, then we have a deficiency in the adrenalin secretion, the driving force that keeps the organs of elimination up and doing their duty.

This condition may be the forerunner of a deficiency in the thyroid hormone, followed by a faulty or a minus metabolism. With this condition at hand we have a perfect setup for arthritis and kindred ailments, and a picture of what we must correct through our reflex work if we are to be successful in rendering a permanent form of relief.

Now if this relief is forthcoming because we have been able to restore the normal harmony of those glands, more power to us, since we will have reached the cause, for up to the present time the use of ACTH is acknowledged to be only a form of temporary ease and not a cure.

Chronic Invalidism

It has been my privilege to double check on cases of chronic invalidism where the cause could not be traced to an abnormal physical condition. Instead it was due to a distorted mental attitude, such as jealousy, hatred, envy, revenge, etc. This had persistently poisoned the system by upsetting the normal glandular secretions, causing discord and inharmony, like that of an orchestra where the instruments are completely out of tune.

I was given an interesting illustration of this not long ago from a member of the medical profession who had become very much interested in what I am teaching. During our discussion of the glands and how our reflex work affected them, etc., he said he had heard the duty of the pituitary gland likened to that of an orchestra leader; the thyroid to the first violinist, etc. If these two important members are at odds with each other, out of tune, causing a discord, what kind of music could we expect from others in the group?

PRIMARY CAUSE

Now where we can prove that the primary cause is a distorted mental attitude, beyond our power to correct or change in any way, I find we might work on the reflexes until doomsday without any results.

CHANGE OF MENTAL ATTITUDE

To change the mental attitude of a patient is not as easy as it might seem, especially with the type who seeks sympathy from some particular source.

The Importance of
Better Care of Our Feet

If people would only realize the importance of taking better care of their feet, we would have less sickness in our land today.

They fail to realize that every corn, callous or bunion, and its location, definitely affects some organ or tissue of the body.

Any undue pressure on a nerve reflex will have a definite effect on the organs involved.

How necessary then that we pay more attention to our feet and visit a chiropodist regularly when any abnormal condition takes place in them.

Terminals

According to our circulatory system the blood is carried from the heart to the terminals of our hands and feet by the arteries. At those points the transfer is made to the veins, which must return that life-giving force to the heart.

Now if these terminals are corroded, if we may use that term, through the lack of normal force supplied from the heart action, over a period of the past, we will improve that vital contact with the electrical forces of the earth obtained under normal conditions, if we can eliminate any foreign substance from the delicate nerve areas.

This is done by a particular form of compression technique scientifically applied to those reflex areas in the feet.

Just how far do we proceed with our automobile if the battery terminals are in any way corroded with a foreign substance?

Hair and Nails

Our nails and hair continue to grow according to the ability of our glands to gather from our food the proper chemicals for their development and growth.

Then is it unreasonable to assume that the pituitary gland may play an important part in causing hair to turn grey prematurely, or baldness to appear?

If anyone is inclined to dispute this assertion and happens to be a subject for demonstration, have him remove his shoe and contact the pituitary gland reflex and see what he will have to say. No doubt he will be ready to accuse you of using your thumbnail or some other sharp object of torture.

I am not holding this out as a remedy, but as a means of stating a most likely cause and a prevention of these abnormal conditions. Perhaps some day someone will find a particular reflex that will do the trick. Here's hoping, but I have not found it as yet.

Hiccoughs

May I call your attention to what may prove of importance to you some day if you are called upon to help a case of hiccoughs.

If nervous tension is the cause, then the proper amount of relaxation will be your success.

It was my privilege to verify this while working in the clinic of the Osteopathic Hospital in St. Petersburg, Florida. An elderly gentleman, over eighty years of age, had been afflicted with them for two years. He had visited numerous hospitals with no permanent relief, but with this form of reflex work I was able to relax the severe tension and correct the condition, even at his advanced age. I found the reflexes to the pituitary, thyroid, prostate glands and solar plexus most tender.

I will relate here an incident that took place in California when the newspapers were giving an account of a severe case. A war worker had been hiccoughing for thirteen days. When reading these articles I expressed my regret that someone trained in the INGHAM COMPRESSION METHOD OF REFLEXOLOGY could not be called to his assistance. A little later I received a letter telling how a Mr. Shope, who had my book *"STORIES THE FEET CAN TELL"* had offered his services and brought relief.

I am copying from the Hospital Corps Quarterly of November, 1944, Vol. 17, No. 6, Page 201, an account of his work and what they had to say about it:

THE PENDLETON SCOUT
B.S. SHOPE, PHM2C, HALTS HICCOUGHS

"To a Camp Pendleton man, B.S. Shope, PhM2c, should go the credit of curing that Los Angeles hiccough victim after days of suffering. Shope turned the trick by what is technically known as Reflexology, even after electric shock treatment failed to effect a permanent cure. The victim, Lawrence Schone, age thirty-one, an aircraft worker, went to sleep for the first time without anaesthetics since his hiccoughs started after Shope worked the man's feet for an hour.

The nerves in the feet are associated with the stomach and diaphragm, Shope explained, and working the nerve reflexes is soothing and relaxing.

The same cure was used by Shope here several months ago, when a Marine fell victim to hiccoughs. Shope effected this cure after the victim hiccoughed two days and two nights.

Reading in the papers about Schone's affliction, Shope offered his services, went to Los Angeles last weekend on his own and treated Schone with the consent of his physician.

Shope worked the victim for an hour. The victim went to sleep, enjoyed his first sound sleep since becoming afflicted. Upon awakening Schone was able to eat his first meal with out hiccoughs returning. Twenty hours later the hiccoughs had not returned, so Schone's physician ordered him released from the hospital. Mrs. Schone and Shope took the patient home, where Shope again worked his feet.

Shope explained that such treatment as electric shock stops hiccoughs for about eight hours, then they start again.

Shope enlisted on September 1, 1942, in Spokane, where he was in physiotherapy at the Sacred Heart Hospital."

Pancreas

The pancreas, termed by some as liver sweetbread, is a gland which must be mentioned respectfully as among the major balancing mechanisms of an individual's metabolism, supplying the blood and lymph with insulin. We must also keep in mind its most immediate antagonists, which are the adrenal glands.

While adrenalin raises the amount of sugar in the blood stream, insulin, whether supplied by the normal function of the gland or administered artificially, will lower it.

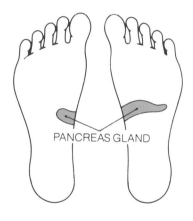

PANCREAS GLAND

71

FIGURE 18

Now we can see and understand why when this compression method is applied to the reflex leading to the adrenal glands and its supply of adrenalin is increased before the condition of the pancreas is normal, we usually find the urine test showing a definite increase of sugar.

This will invariably happen, together with our ability to increase the activity of the liver, which, even normally, is always in readiness to supply extra sugar to the blood stream to produce energy in cases of emergency.

Diabetes

For obtaining results in a case of diabetes, follow what I have said on this subject in my book,*"STORIES THE FEET CAN TELL,"* with the additional suggestions I am giving you in this chapter.

Look for trouble in the other gland reflexes, especially the pituitary and thyroid glands.

True diabetes is due to an insufficient amount of insulin, a hormone that is normally produced by the pancreatic gland, the function of which is to prevent a defective metabolism of the sugars and starches of our food.

IF CAUSED BY SHOCK OR GRIEF

You have all seen cases of diabetes where the primary cause could be traced to some definite shock or grief that had affected the entire glandular system.

These cases will usually respond to this reflex method which definitely corrects the excessive nervous tension brought on by shock or grief. They will not, however, require so many treatments.

If such patients are already taking insulin, they must be warned what to do when the pancreatic gland begins to throw a normal supply of insulin directly into the blood stream in addition to what is being taken hypodermically. Then the same procedure must be followed as that which would be used for insulin shock for which their physicians would recommend an immediate intake of additional sugar.

EDUCATE THE PATIENT

When the patient has been educated to this effect, he will realize that this reaction is true to form. He will not be worried at this increase of sugar showing up in the urine test.

Instead it will increase his faith in what you are able to do. He can then be led to believe that your work is doing something to help nature dispel the excessive sugar from the liver and kidneys.

When this has been accomplished, after the first few treatments, that condition will disappear and you will begin to see a definite improvement following each application of this compression technique. You will have worked on the reflex to each of the important glands where any tenderness was found to exist and in so doing you will have corrected the primary cause.

These statements will be verified to your own satisfaction after trying this INGHAM COMPRESSION METHOD OF REFLEXOLOGY on a few of your patients.

DIABETES IN CHILDREN

I hesitate to offer much encouragement for relieving a diabetic condition in children.

Often in such cases I have learned upon questioning the mother that she recalled some shock or grief which had occurred during her pregnancy. The question then arises as to whether this condition could have had any effect on the glands of the unborn child and could have been a contributing factor in the development of diabetes in the child after birth.

Let me leave this question with you as food for thought, for we are being told today that infants can catch fear and hatred from those around them more quickly than they can catch measles or any other infectious disease.

Kidney Stones

Would stones in the kidneys exist if the normal chemistry of the blood stream were sustained?

We are told that one in every five persons suffers from kidney stones. If a patient has been diagnosed as having kidney stones and it has been verified by X-ray, etc., then your endeavor is to create sufficient relaxation to pass those stones through the urinary tract.

You want to improve the muscle tone of the ureter, which is the excretory duct leading from the kidney to the bladder, a tube having a muscular coating and comparable in size to a goose quill, about fourteen to sixteen inches long, extending from the kidney to the base of the bladder. See Fig. 19.

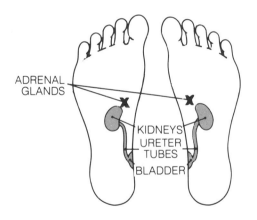

ADRENAL GLANDS

KIDNEYS
URETER
TUBES
BLADDER

FIGURE 19

FILTRATION PLANT

As a delicate filtration plant, the kidneys have two different functions to perform. They must separate certain elements necessary for health, then build the muscle tone required to throw off the poisonous waste matter.

The muscle tone for this will be built up and furnished mainly by the secretion of adrenalin sent out by the adrenal glands. They in turn await their orders from the thyroid and pituitary glands.

When any one of this gland family becomes sluggish and indolent, the others suffer in proportion in their duty. The normal contraction and relaxation of these glands will have lost a certain degree of muscle tone which the INGHAM COMPRESSION METHOD OF REFLEXOLOGY endeavors to restore by its particular contact with the nerve impulses whose terminals are in the feet.

This work has proved its effect on the highly sensitive sympathetic nervous system governing the functions of the involuntary organs of our body.

Kidney Action

If the kidneys are overactive, causing too frequent urination, you must bring this condition back to normal. If they are abnormally inactive, failing to contract and relax as nature intended, you must correct this and bring the kidney action up to normal.

Remember nature's tendency is to normalize, correct and restore any abnormal condition that may exist when we give her the necessary material (circulation) with which to rebuild any sick broken-down gland or organ of the body.

It is most important to remember how the action of the kidney is controlled by the involuntary nervous system and how the involuntary nervous system is controlled by the highly sensitive sympathetic nerves. Therefore, you can readily understand why an emotional upset could produce an irregularity in kidney action, verifying the fact that stress or distress, also fright, anger, etc., can have a definite effect in the function of urination.

By keeping this in mind it is easy to understand why these conditions so often respond readily when we have relaxed the excessive nervous tension set up in the solar plexus. See Fig 9, pg. 39.

Our brain is the nucleus of the muscular system, a reliable dispenser of information.

Our body is one unit, the solar plexus being considered the psychic center, governing the subconscious mind and the involuntary activities of our being.

CASE HISTORY

One day in Miami, Florida, a prominent physician came to see me, with an open mind, to investigate what I had to offer.

We were doing some extensive research work at that time in the field of reflex work to verify the accuracy of these reflexes in the feet and their relationship according to the principles of ZONE THERAPY.

As I proceeded with a careful examination of his feet I found the reflex to his right kidney very tender, while the reflex to his left kidney showed no tenderness whatever, telling me the story that I had encountered an unusual condition.

He being a physician familiar with this INGHAM COMPRESSION METHOD OF REFLEXOLOGY we discussed freely what these findings revealed, that definitely some abnormal condition existed with the right kidney. It was failing to contract and relax as nature intended, allowing congestion to form in that particular reflex area, while that of the left kidney, which apparently was functioning normally, showed no tenderness whatever.

The physician then verified my findings by telling how at the age of four years he was taken seriously ill with Bright's Disease. The doctors, seeing no hope, gave him forty-eight hours to live, but his mother saved his life by giving him some old-fashioned remedy. Later diagnosis had pronounced it to be an inactive kidney on the right side and he had been advised at various times to have it removed.

High Blood Pressure

Let us remember a patient who has high blood pressure is not being treated for high blood pressure, but for the condition responsible for it.

High blood pressure is not a disease in itself, rather it is the effect or result of an underlying abnormal condition. It may be faulty elimination, which could result from some deficiency of the glandular system, especially the adrenal glands. It is their special duty to supply the system with sufficient adrenalin to normalize the circulatory system, so important in maintaining the proper chemical balance.

If the blood stream contains an abnormal amount of calcium, it will adhere to the walls of the arteries and blood vessels so they no longer retain their normal elasticity, increasing the effort of the heart in performing its special duty.

Hypertension must be considered an important factor when seeking to relieve high blood pressure.

Remember, the proper balance between digestion and elimination cannot be obtained where undue tension exists. When we can remove this tension then a balanced functioning of all the organs may be restored if they have not reached an irreversible state. Nature is a true healing power but only from within can she repair damaged or diseased tissues by the building material produced through circulation not impeded by tension often found following a distorted mental attitude. There in no higher goal for us in life than to keep improving the health and happiness of our fellow men.

Atrophy of the Optic Nerve

While in California last year we had the privilege of testing the efficiency of the INGHAM COMPRESSION METHOD OF REFLEXOLOGY in connection with a case diagnosed by the medical profession as atrophy of the optic nerve.

Mrs. C., whose husband had been associated with the U.S. Navy for a number of years, had been attended by the best specialists throughout the country, who could offer no help for her condition. She had been told that even her ability to distinguish shadows would last but a little longer, yet she had a smile and a happy mental attitude I shall never forget. She was taking up a study of Braille and refused to worry and poison her system with fear and anxiety over the dark outlook facing her at that time.

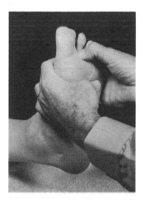

FIGURE 20
Position for Working the Reflex to the Eyes.

She was unable to distinguish any color, due to what appeared to be a dense fog before her eyes. We sought to find the cause before we could hope to relieve the effect.

We found the reflexes to the kidneys and adrenal glands very tender. Keeping in mind how closely associated the functioning of the kidneys appears to be with many an abnormal condition of the eyes, it was easy to assume they might be a contributing factor in this case.

We then proceeded to contact the reflex to the area relative to the back of the neck, to see if any part of the normal blood supply to the head and eyes was being cut off. From the tenderness we discovered we could read another definite chapter into our story of investigation.

After some questioning we learned Mrs. C. had an automobile accident a few years prior to this condition now affecting her eyes.

Three weeks later, after our persistent work on those tender reflexes, she was able to distinguish colors. She could work in her flower garden and determine the difference between roses and sweet peas. She read the advertising signs as we drove along the road. Recently she wrote me a splendid letter telling of her recovery.

Apoplexy

We are all familiar with the effect of emotions and the part they play in raising the blood pressure of a highly emotional individual. It is when he is aroused suddenly by some extreme circumstance that the pressure rises to a point beyond what the blood vessels in the brain can withstand and he has an apoplectic stroke.

This condition is caused by an acute vascular lesion of the brain, resulting in hemorrhage, thrombosis or embolism, and followed by paralysis.

The location of this lesion determines the side which will be paralyzed. If the *left* side of the body is paralyzed, the *right* side of the brain will be involved, and vice versa. We, therefore, must look to the reflex in the *right* big toe for the proper point of contact with the reflex to the *right* side of the brain. If the *right* side of the body is paralyzed, we must look to the reflex in the *left* big toe to help relieve the excessive tension in the *left* side of the brain where the embolism took place.

The crossing of certain nerve impulses has no relationship with the reflexes. For a reflex contact with the right eye, we look to the eye reflex in the right foot; for the left eye, the reflex in the left foot. The first, second, third, fourth and fifth zones of the right side of the head are related to the same zones in the right big toe. The left side of the head is similarly related to the left big toe.

Circulation

The blood leaves the heart by the aorta, the largest of the arteries on the left side of the heart.

The arteries are spread throughout the trunk of the body and are thick-walled, elastic vessels, which carry the blood away from the heart. They divide and subdivide, increasing in number and decreasing in size, until they become the tiny capillaries in all the tissues of the body, disposed in the form of a network.

Through the membranous walls of the capillaries oxygen and carbon dioxide are exchanged between the tissues and the blood. Through these same walls food is given to the tissues and waste products are returned to the blood, if metabolism is properly balanced. But if the blood circulation in any area is inadequate, from the result of hypertension, the waste matter (end products) is not completely eliminated.

The capillaries finally merge or combine to form the veins through which the blood is then returned to the heart. The veins grow larger and larger as they approach the heart, until the two largest, known as the superior and inferior vena cava, empty into the right auricle of the heart, on the right side of the heart. Here the venous blood is sent through the lungs to be purified, returns to the left side of the heart and repeats its journey through the body.

In the arteries the blood flows rapidly; in the capillaries it oozes along sluggishly; and in the veins flows at a more rapid rate as it approaches the heart.

A REAL PICTURE

Now you have a picture in mind as to how the blood, through its marvelous circulatory system, makes a definite transfer from the arteries to the veins in the area of those extremities (reflexes) in the hands and feet.

This process is carried on by a contraction and relaxation rhythm, normally timed by nature to an exact point, to prevent any delay in the normal transmission of the blood from the arteries to the veins.

Who could fail to believe that such a delicate set-up cannot be disrupted by mental stress and hypertension?

Epilepsy

Epilepsy, like migraine, is usually a nervous symptom and from recent reports backed by medical authority we learn it can often be linked to, or associated with, some form of allergy—a symptom of allergic reaction. With this in mind we can readily understand why we have been successful in so many cases in giving relief to those afflicted with this malady.

If we can normalize the chemical reaction of the glands of internal secretion, correcting any abnormal acid or alkaline balance of the mucous membrane of the alimentary canal, the respiratory tract and its many branches, will we not lessen the susceptibility to epilepsy, migraine, asthma, hay fever, hives, eczema, or any of the numerous disorders whose origin can be traced to some form of allergy?

It is the opinion of some who have made a special study of this condition that eighty-five per cent of those suffering from epilepsy were found to have a faulty colon. Even many of our so-called colds of today are considered to have an allergic basis caused by an oversensitive colon.

With this thought in mind let me ask you to try out carefully all the various reflexes to determine *which* one may show the *greatest* degree of tenderness. This will give you a lead as to where the condition may originate, whether it may be coming from a faulty colon, some form of allergy, or the result of some glandular disturbance.

To a physician who is licensed to diagnose and depends upon the administration of drugs for his results, this work can prove most valuable, for in his work a correct diagnosis is the most important factor, so he can make sure what is best to prescribe. But those who are not licensed to diagnose or prescribe and are dependent upon drugless methods only for their results, *must* learn to refrain from telling the patient what they find to be affected. They will proceed to use this INGHAM COMPRESSION METHOD OF REFLEXOLOGY to break up the congestion and relieve tension in the nerve reflex to whatever gland or organ of the body may be at fault.

Lymph Glands

The lymph we find to be a form of blood serum supplied by the lymph glands, a most vital life-giving fluid. It is transparent, a slightly yellow liquid, having an alkaline reaction.

Following its course are small seed-like enlargements, little knots, which play an active part in destroying infection. A good many of these we find in the neck as nature's safeguard to control any infection of the teeth, tonsils, etc. Also we find a liberal supply of these seed-like knots under the armpits and in the groin, serving as a wall of resistance for any infection that may invade the extremities, hands, feet, etc.

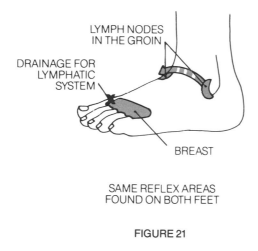

LYMPH NODES IN THE GROIN

DRAINAGE FOR LYMPHATIC SYSTEM

BREAST

SAME REFLEX AREAS FOUND ON BOTH FEET

FIGURE 21

If there is any cause to believe these glands are failing to do the work allotted to them by nature, then in addition to your working on the other gland reflexes I want you to use a heavy deep movement around the ankle bone on top of the foot.

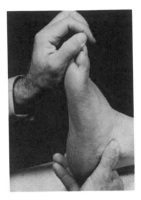

FIGURE 22

**Position of the Thumb for Working Reflex
to the Lymph Glands Relative to Groin and
Armpits (Both Feet).**

If you find a tenderness in that location it is telling you a story these glands need attention. Get busy, work it out and watch for results.

Breast

We are often asked where the reflex area to the breast may be found. As you examine cut above you will see where we are calling your attention to the reflex to the lymph glands in the groin and armpits. With this picture in mind follow down to the roots of the toes over the top of the foot, in the same corresponding zone as that where the trouble is found in the breast. See Fig. 21.

Parathyroid Glands

The four parathyroid glands, each comparing in size to a kernel of wheat, lie close against the thyroid gland.

They govern the calcium content of the blood stream, having close relationship to bone metabolism—bone tissue change. Thus any method of improving a thyroid disturbance would definitely aid in correcting a faulty functioning of the parathyroids.

Do not let these tiny glands make the mistake of sending too much of the calcium content of the blood stream into the muscle tissue instead of the bony structure of the body.

Keep this in mind when you find a rheumatic or arthritic condition, accompanied by ankylosis, which tells you the story that there is an over-supply of calcium, wrongly distributed throughout the system.

When this oversupply of calcium content is deposited in the muscle tissue the resulting condition will be diagnosed as rheumatism; when it is found deposited in the joints it will be diagnosed as arthritis.

Asthma

We are familiar with the distress and suffering experienced by those who are afflicted with asthma and hay fever. Today this is acknowledged to be a form of allergy, the symptoms of which depend on the inherent susceptibility of the individual.

It is the abnormal chemical balance of the mucous membrane of the nose and throat. This furnishes a fertile field for the irritating effect of pollen, which may come from tree or plant, causing one to sneeze and sniff because of the mucous membrane irritation.

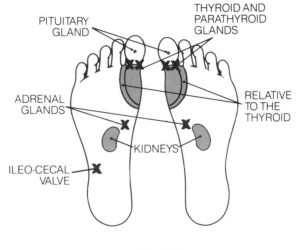

FIGURE 23

It will cause the eyes to water, for this pollen is likened to a cinder which the eyes are endeavoring to clear away.

POLLEN

In 1880 a scientist by the name of Charles Blackley first discovered the effect of pollen on the mucous membrane of the eyes, nose and throat and its effect in causing them to become swollen and inflamed, yet having no effect on the outer layer of the skin, which is composed of dead nonreactive tissue.

Between the trees, grasses, and last but not least, the weeds, we have three distinct hay fever seasons in the United States; one in the spring from tree pollen, one in summer from grasses, and one in the autumn from weeds, which far exceeds the others in the amount of misery it can cause.

Lucretius of the first century B.C., gave us the adage, "What is food to one man, may be poison to another," a concise description of food allergy.

All that is new about the word allergy is the name, for the symptoms have been known for a long, long, time. Allergy is a sensitiveness to our environment.

Dr. Bree in 1800 wrote a treatise on asthma in which he described it as "A convulsive attempt on the part of the respiratory organs to remove some sort of irritation arising either in the lungs or in some closely related viscera."

HORMONES RELATING TO ASTHMA AND HAY FEVER

A hormone is a chemical substance produced normally in the various glands of the body. The hormone adrenalin is considered most important in the cause of, and the treatment for, asthma. A deficiency in this specific hormone produced by the adrenal glands is what we find when a patient is suffering from a form of allergy known as asthma.

Let me entreat you to give special attention to the adrenal gland reflexes in any case of asthma or hay fever you are trying to relieve. Apply the INGHAM COMPRESSION METHOD OF REFLEXOLOGY to stimulate the action of these important glands when you see there is a deficiency in the normal production of this important hormone substance, which is leaving the patient susceptible not only to asthma, but also hay fever.

We are told sixty per cent of the inadequately treated hay fever victims become asthmatics, some of whom may be doomed to a life of invalidism. These effects may be a protective protest by nature against the offending cause in which the whole body is capable of participating.

Allergy may be a general reaction manifesting itself anywhere in the body where mucous membrane, or smooth muscle tissue, is found to exist, but naturally affecting first the nose, throat, bronchial area, etc., which has received primary attention, due to the ability of that area to register the loudest protest.

CASE HISTORY

You will be interested in hearing what this work did for a little boy seven years old in St. Petersburg, Florida, who suffered with asthma since he was a year and a half old.

Numerous methods and remedies, costing thousands of dollars, had failed to give more than a slight degree of relief. From allergy tests he had been considered allergic to wheat and forbidden to eat any wheat products whatever. Despite the fact that his parents adhered strictly to these orders the boy still suffered constantly with attacks of asthma and hay fever.

As I took his feet in my hands and proceeded to see WHAT STORIES THEY COULD BE MADE TO TELL I soon found I had an unusual case before me. Here was a child of seven with every gland reflex showing an extremely high degree of tenderness, with the adrenal gland reflexes in the lead, true to form, showing the greatest degree of tenderness. Next came the thyroid, the pituitary, the prostate, and last but not least, the ileocecal valve reflex showed a definite degree of sensitiveness. See Fig. 23 Pg. 88.

It was on January 27th when we began to work on these tender areas, alternating from one to the other for about fifteen to twenty minutes all told at each visit not more often than twice a week. By May 10th the tenderness had been practically worked out. He had gained twelve pounds, was eating, playing and doing everything the same as any other child his age, with no more asthma attacks, regardless of what he ate or did.

Does this not prove again that the tendency to or the cause of an allergy can often be traced to a deficiency of the hormone supply, due to a faulty functioning of the glandular system?

Can we imagine anything of more importance than to be able to relax the undue tension of these important life-giving glands?

CASE HISTORY

Learn the right thing to do, and know how to do it right. Then as we grow in the scientific knowledge of these reflex methods our ability and efficiency will increase.

Another strikingly interesting case is that of my husband. Mr. Stopfel came to me as a patient in 1941, having heard of my work and what I had accomplished for others in his condition who were suffering with asthma.

For over forty years he had been considered a most extreme case of both asthma and hay fever, which followed an attack of scarlet fever when he was nine years old. Nothing he had done heretofore had afforded more than temporary relief.

After listening to the history of his case, I proceeded to look for WHAT STORIES HIS FEET COULD BE MADE TO TELL, what gland reflexes would be found tender as the result of asthma in his particular case.

Now unlike that of the little boy in Florida I did not find every gland reflex tender, but instead it seemed to be confined to the adrenal first and the thyroid second. Why do I say the adrenal first and the thyroid second? Because the reflexes to the adrenal gland showed a greater degree of tenderness than the reflexes to the thyroid gland. The pituitary seemed to take third place in his particular case. After verifying this to my own satisfaction I then contacted the reflex to the ileocecal valve. It, too, was very tender, telling me in no uncertain terms that the mucous from the small intestines was not being normally eliminated through the intestinal tract, leaving an excessive amount of this to be taken care of through the respiratory organs.

After relaxing the nervous tension set up by this long standing asthmatic condition, I had accomplished a great deal toward ultimate relief. I had improved the contraction and relaxation of his diaphragm, another important area in a case of this type. He began gradually to improve. As his vitality increased his fear of those dreaded attacks decreased and it can truthfully be said he has been entirely free of them ever since, regardless of many severe tests. Let me relate one instance I distinctly recall which followed the completion of my reflex work on his feet, after all the congestion and tenderness had been worked out.

We were on our way driving home from California, crossing the desert one hot afternoon in August when the temperature must have registered over one hundred degrees. There in the midst of a field of goldenrod and dust a tire went down, requiring him to make the change under those extreme conditions. After completing the task without even a sneeze he assured me that the INGHAM COMPRESSION METHOD OF REFLEXOLOGY could certainly do wonders for asthma, regardless of how severe or of how long standing it may have been.

To Blaze the Path

If it has been allotted to me to blaze the path of some new discovery, I hope I will accept it as a gift from GOD placed in my hands, my heart and my soul, and may I never be puzzled because of opposition. Many before me have given their lives to an ideal, to a cause and after having left this earthly scene, others have come along and lifted the torch. If any obstacle should beset our path through disbelief on the part of those inclined to be skeptical, remember, our ability to pass over it will only strengthen our faith in what we have proven to be true. Centuries ago, King Solomon, in addressing his people, spoke with the same sentiment, "There is no new thing under the sun."

To substantiate the principles I have outlined in my two books of which some readers may still be skeptical, I have recently found in my research, further evidence of this theory written as far back as 1846 in a book, *"Therapeutic Sarcognomy (Science of the Soul, Brain and Body)."*

Excerpts from "THERAPEUTIC SARCOGNOMY"
By
JOSEPH BUCHANAN, M.D.

Dr. Joseph Buchanan was Professor of Physiology in four Medical Colleges successively from 1846 to 1881.

QUOTE:

"The reader should understand that each portion of the surface of the body is related directly to a physiological function through its sympathetic connection with the psychic organ, the brain. The map of the organs of the BRAIN is reproduced on the body.

This wonderful discovery made in 1842 has been verified in innumerable experiments since by myself and my pupils and being a law of nature in verified in every disease.

Its demonstration is so easy and convincing that the science will be universally recognized as the most important addition ever made to biology as soon as the attention of the educated is seriously given the investigation, for all competent and candid observers will easily find what I have found and what all my pupils readily discover in others and in themselves.

From page 644:
Intense stimulation of the lower limbs has great power to arouse the dormant vitality of the base of the brain.

The relation of the lower limbs to the brain is not realized by physicians generally as it should be to enable them to relieve the head and chest.

From page 645:
Dr. H.W. Green of Kentucky reports a severe and protracted case of epilepsy in a Negro defying all medical treatment, which was suspended, after he fell in a fit and *burned badly* the *whole* of the bottom of the foot. During the four months his fits ceased and his health was good, but the fits returned after the foot was healed.

The ease with which experiments upon the brain and the body may be made by any intelligent person according to my methods and the innumerable illustrations of *"Therapeutic Sarcognomy (Science of the Soul, Brain and Body)"* observable in disease, will make the subject so clear to intelligent inquirers that the wonder will be hereafter how anything so plain and so accessible could have been so long overlooked and its first scientific announcement received with such absent-minded indifference, owing to the mental perversions of the false education and the self-satisfied enjoyment of old theories, with a thoughtless unconsciousness of the vast realms of knowledge upon which mankind are slowly entering.

From page 633:
"How few are the men (says Dr. Ashburner) who acquire gouty habits, who do not lose the power of calm reasoning. They are notoriously an irritable race. Their irritability often leads them to conclude that everyone is wrong except themselves. No matter if you can bring abundant evidence to prove the insanity of their conduct, it is of no avail."

Dr. J.A. Roberts reported in the "Eclectic Medical Journal" of October, 1887, a case of swelling in the thyroid and parotid gland, accompanied by a painful swollen knee, which reproduced a sullen, crabbed state of mind, so that "he could scarcely speak, unless asked a question, but after opening the gland, discharging its pus and aspiration four ounces of fluid from the knee, he "became quite talkative," and "anything I wished was cheerfully granted."

Pain is itself an irritating element, but in other parts of the body it may be accompanied by fortitude or resignation; but in the foot, which is the site of the first attack of gout, the unreasoning or anti-cerebral character of the foot. This local disturbance deranges the balance even of strong constitutions; but if we would realize fully the character which Sarcognomy recognizes in each spot, we must have a constitution sufficiently weak, sensitive and impressible to surrender to the control of the local excitement. In such a case the mind may be entirely perverted by an irritation in the feet, as in a case reported by Dr. Anderson of idiocy and violence produced by an injury of the foot and the tibial nerve the irritation of which extended up to the thigh. Dr. James Anderson of New York reported in the N.Y. Medical and Physical Journal of which extended up to the thigh. Dr. James Anderson of New York reported in the N.Y. Medical and Physical Journal of December, 1822, a case of prostration of the intellect from an injury of the foot affecting the anterior tibial nerve.

From page 664:
A lad, age 14, as he was getting up in the morning, was heard by his father to be making a great noise in his bedroom. As the latter rushed into the room he found his son in his shirt violently agitated, talking incoherently and breaking to pieces the furniture. His father caught hold of him and put him back into bed when at once the boy became composed but did not seem at all conscious of what he had done. On getting out of bed he had felt "somewhat odd" he said, but he was quite well. A surgeon who was sent for, found him still reading quietly with a clean tongue and cheerful countenance and wishful to get up. He had never had epilepsy, but had enjoyed good health hitherto.

He was told to get up, but on putting his foot on the floor and standing up, his countenance changed, the jaw became instantly convulsed, and he was about to rush forward when he was seized and pushed back into the bed. At once he became calm again, said he had "felt odd," but surprised when asked what was the matter with him. He had been fishing on the previous day, and having got his line entangled had waded into the river to disengage it, but was not aware that he had hurt his feet in any way or that he had ever scratched them.

But in holding up the right great toe with my finger and thumb to examine the sole of the foot, the leg was drawn up and the muscles of the jaw were suddenly convulsed, and on letting go the toe these effects instantly ceased. There was no redness nor swelling, but in the BULB OF THE TOE a small elevation as if a bit of gravel, less than the head of a pin, had been pressed beneath the cuticle. On compressing this against the nail cautiously, a slight convulsion ensued. There was no pain when pressed, but he said something made him feel very odd. The slightly raised part was clipped away, no gravel was found, but the strange sensation was gone and never returned.

Here I must pause in this hasty pathological illustration of Sarcognomy, although the theme is not half exhausted. Time does not permit a fuller exposition at present.

To those who do not know the absolute certainty of Sarcognomy as a science and have made no experiments for its illustration it is probable that the facts of pathology may be useful in relieving them from the feeling of uncertainty which embarrasses the approach to a new and revolutionary science.

This work I hope may be the means of stimulating the SINCERE and FEARLESS leaders of beneficient science to explore still farther the boundless realm to which it has opened the way, which will be enjoyed by thousands, when the hand that pens these lines shall have vanished from earthly scenes."

End Quote.

In Conclusion

This work as I am presenting it in my books and seminars, has grown to a high state of recognition and acceptance at a rate beyond what any of you realize unless permitted to read the letters we receive daily from coast to coast and from many foreign countries to which my books have been mailed. May we continue to offer this special contribution to the public (the laymen and the profession) for their health and well being, not as a cure but as a valuable asset to avenues of relief. We know the practice of this Science is in no way deleterious to the human body.

Green Pastures

We are so prone to feel that what is wrong in our lives is not ourselves, but in the external setting of our lives.

Dr. Fosdick said in a radio sermon, "Not all the water in the seven seas can sink a ship unless it gets inside."

It is from within, the desire we have to get well in terms of *hope, vision* and *courage,* that will influence the functioning of our glands.

We try to fool ourselves and place the blame for our illness on external things, on the pastures where we happen to be feeding. Instead, it is what we cause to happen in the functioning of our glands within the body, through the type of thinking we have done, that will make the pastures grow greener; and not something on the outside, barring accident.

Let us then look for the green pastures right where we live, move and have our being. For the green pastures are within ourselves, in our way of thinking, our mode of life. These are the green pastures where David the psalmist said, "He maketh me to lie down."

That continued success may attend your efforts, both now and in the years to follow, is my sincere desire.

Faithfully yours,

EUNICE INGHAM STOPFEL